THE
TRUTH ABOUT OPIUM-SMOKING

STATED BY

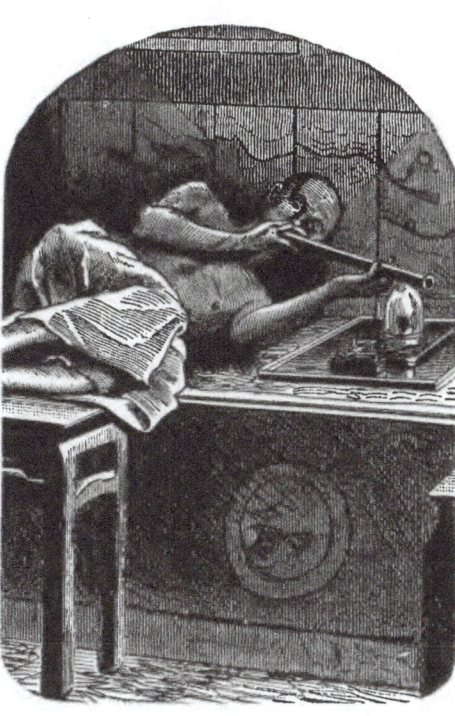

MISSIONARIES.

Rev. F. W. BALLER.
Rev. W. H. COLLINS.
Dr. GALT.
Dr. GAULD.
Rev. D. HILL.
Rev. G. JOHN.
Dr. MAXWELL.
Rev. J. MCCARTHY.
Rev. A. E. MOULE.
Rev. J. SADLER.

BRITISH OFFICIALS.

Sir R. ALCOCK,
Sir THOMAS WADE,
AND OTHERS.

CHINESE OFFICIALS.

LI HUNG-CHANG,
WEN-SEANG,
AND OTHERS.

ARCHBISHOPS:
CANTERBURY, YORK.
BISHOPS;
MEMBERS OF
PARLIAMENT, AND
OTHERS.

With Illustrations.

LONDON:
HODDER & STOUGHTON, PATERNOSTER ROW.
1882.

CONTENTS.

---o---

	PAGES
INTRODUCTION,	5–16
PROCEEDINGS AT CONFERENCE ON OPIUM-SMOKING,	17–30

    Speakers.—Lord Polwarth (chairman); Rev. W. H. Collins, M.R.C.S.; Dr. Gauld; Dr. Maxwell; Dr. Galt; Rev. A. E. Moule; Rev. J. Sadler, and others.

PROCEEDINGS AT PUBLIC MEETING ON OPIUM-SMOKING.

Testimony of Rev. David Hill,	31
Sixteen years missionary in China.	
Testimony of Rev. Arthur E. Moule, B.D.,	34
Twenty-one years missionary in China.	
Testimony of Dr. Gauld,	37
Sixteen years medical missionary in China.	
Testimony of J. Galt, Esq., M.R.C.S.E.,	40
Formerly in charge of the Church Missionary Society's Opium Hospital at Hang-chow.	
Testimony of Rev. F. W. Baller,	42
Eight years missionary in China.	
Testimony of Rev. W. H. Collins, M.R.C.S.,	44
Twenty-three years medical missionary in China.	
Testimony of Rev. James Sadler,	46
Sixteen years missionary to the Chinese.	
Speech of Lord Polwarth,	48
,, Mr. Donald Matheson,	50
,, Mr. T. A. Denny,	50
,, Rev. J. McCarthy,	52
Testimony of Dr. Maxwell,	52
Eight years medical missionary in China.	
Testimony of Rev. J. McCarthy,	56
Twelve years missionary in China.	
Testimony of Rev. Griffith John,	61
Twenty-six years missionary in China.	

APPENDIX.

                                                                          PAGE

ANSWERS TO EXCUSES FOR THE OPIUM TRADE.

    Excuse 1. *Opium-smoking not very injurious,* . . . 65
        Testimony of the Chinese—British Officials—Medical Men.

    Excuse 2. *The Chinese not sincere in their desire to suppress opium-smoking,* 75
        Testimony of Sir Rutherford Alcock—Li Hung-chang—the Chinese—Growth of opium in China no proof of insincerity—Testimony of Sir Rutherford Alcock and others.

    Excuse 3. *The British Government has not forced China to admit opium,* 81
        Testimony of Sir Rutherford Alcock—Commissioner Kwei-lang—Sir Thomas Wade—Lord Elgin—Rev. H. Grattan Guinness—Sir Edward Fry—Rev. James Johnston.

    Excuse 4. *If opium was forced upon China, we are not responsible for what others did long ago,* . . 85
        Sir Edward Fry—Rev. A. S. Thelwall, M.A.

    Excuse 5. *If we do not send opium to China, others will,* . 86

    Excuse 6. *That opium-smoking in China is not worse than intoxicating drink in England,* . . 86

THE OPIUM MONOPOLY, ... 87
    A proposal; very candid, if not very wise—A larger revenue with less labour—An erroneous issue.

THE OPIUM TRADE AND BRITISH COMMERCE, . . . 89
    Injurious to British Commerce, by David M'Laren, Esq.—Cotton Goods and the Opium Trade—Rev. Goodeve Mabbs—London Bankers on the Opium Trade—Mr. S. Manders—Dr. Dudgeon.

THE OPIUM TRADE AS NOW CARRIED ON A NATIONAL SIN, WHICH MUST BRING RETRIBUTION, ... 94
    Dr. Norman Macleod—Sir Arthur Cotton—The late M'Leod Wylie, Esq.—Cardinal Manning.

PROTEST OF THE LATE R. MONTGOMERY MARTIN, ESQ., . 97

LETTER FROM SIR ARTHUR COTTON, ... 99

IMPORTANT TESTIMONIES, ... 102
    Archbishop of Canterbury—Archbishop of York—Bishop of Madras—Earl of Shaftesbury—The late Dr. Punshon—Mr. Henry Richards, M.P.

PARLIAMENTARY ACTION, ... 106
    Sir J. W. Pease's Notice of Motion—Letters from the Archbishop of York—The Bishop of Durham—The Bishop of Liverpool—The Bishop of Exeter.

SIGNS OF PROGRESS IN PUBLIC ENLIGHTENMENT, . . 108

ILLUSTRATIONS.

An Opium-Smoker,	30
Li Hung-chang,	64
Chinese Officials—Prince Kung and Wen-seang,	67
The Poppy,	79
Chinese Merchants,	91
The Opium-Smoker—No. 1,	113
The Opium-Smoker—No. 2,	114
The Opium-Smoker—No. 3,	115
The Opium-Smoker—No. 4,	116

INTRODUCTION.

The following pages will, it is believed, prove valuable to those who desire to form a sound judgment on some disputed points in the controversy on the opium question.

That controversy is rapidly becoming one of the foremost questions of the day, and the nature and magnitude of the interests involved, both moral and material, will, now that the issues have been fairly raised, secure for it henceforth a continually increasing measure of public attention until satisfactorily settled.

Twenty, thirty, forty and more years ago, there were those who earnestly protested against England's connection with the opium trade as then carried on with China. Their efforts to arouse public attention seemed unavailing. Few apparently gave heed.

It is otherwise now. Motions in Parliament, resolutions adopted in Convocation, in Church Congresses, Wesleyan Conferences, Congregational and Baptist Unions, and in public meetings all over the country, condemnatory of England's connection with the opium trade, are so many indications of the awakening of the public conscience to the national sin committed by England in forcing the Government of China to admit our Indian opium.

The meeting at the Mansion House, presided over by the Lord Mayor, and at which the Archbishop of Canterbury, Cardinal Manning, Rev. E. E. Jenkins, ex-President of the Wesleyan Conference, and the Earl of Shaftesbury were among the speakers, was a notable evidence of public feeling upon the question.

With such signs of progress multiplying on every hand, it was becoming manifest that the opium revenue was doomed, when almost simultaneously, and not without indications that they were acting in concert, a number of gentlemen came forward to justify the use of opium, and to vindicate the morality of the opium revenue. Their appearance was as unexpected as their arguments were strange.

Foremost among these was Sir Rutherford Alcock, the man who of all others had done most to furnish material for the anti-opium agitation.

A few days later Sir George Birdwood, in a letter which appeared in the *Times* of Dec. 6, 1881, made the startling announcement that opium-smoking was 'absolutely harmless,' 'almost as harmless an indulgence as twiddling the thumbs.' The following are his own words:—

> 'As regards opium-smoking, I can from experience testify that it is of itself absolutely harmless.'
>
> ... 'I repeat that, of itself, opium-smoking is almost as harmless an indulgence as twiddling the thumbs and other silly-looking methods for concentrating the jaded mind.
>
> ... '*All I insist on is the downright innocency, in itself, of opium-smoking; and that, therefore,* so far as we are concerned in its morality, whether judged by a standard based on a deduction from preconceived religious ideas, or an induction from national practices, *we are as free to introduce opium into China, and to raise a revenue from it in India, as to export our cotton, iron, and woollen manufactures to France.*
>
> 'I am not approving the use of stimulants—I have long ceased to do so. I am only protesting that there is no more harm in smoking opium than in smoking tobacco in the form of the mildest cigarettes, and that its narcotic effect can be but infinitesimal —if, indeed, anything measurable; and I feel bound to publicly express these convictions, which can easily be put to the test of experiment, at a moment when all the stupendous machinery available in this country of crotchet-mongers and ignorant if well-meaning agitators, is being set in movement against the Indian opium revenue on the express ground of its falsely imputed immorality.'

Such statements, coming though they did from one who in some subjects had a well-earned reputation, were looked upon as too absurd to do any harm, and as not worthy of serious reply. It soon became apparent, however, that their circulation in the *Times* had given them an adventitious importance, and in various parts of the country many who had read them were greatly perplexed. It seemed to them improbable that a man who had any professional reputation to lose, would so trifle with it as to make, with such iteration, statements so definite and positive, unless he had some foundation in fact for his assertions.

Deputy-Surgeon-General Moore was another who came forward, 'actuated,' he said, 'by the firm impression that the British public were being misled by probably well-meaning but certainly mistaken persons.' He thought it unlikely that the people of England would consent to all that the loss of the opium revenue would involve;

> 'especially when they would be doing so for the purpose of preventing a comparatively few Chinamen suffering from the abuse of an agent which many more Chinamen find to be a source of enjoyment, of comfort, a necessity, and even a blessing.'

These views Dr. Moore sought to justify.

Another apologist for opium-smoking appeared in the person of a Mr. Brereton, a solicitor from Hong-Kong. In a public lecture he said:

> 'I had daily intercourse with the people, from whom the best and truest information on the subject of opium can be obtained, and my experience is, that opium-smoking, as practised in China, is perfectly innocuous.'

And he asserted that of all the British residents in China not one per cent. could be found

> 'who will not declare that opium-smoking in China is a harmless, if not an absolutely beneficial practice; that it produces no decadence in mind or body; and that the allegations as to its demoralizing effects are simply ridiculous.'

He even said:

> 'I have tried to find the victims of the dreadful drug, but I have never yet succeeded.'

Sir George Birdwood, Dr. Moore, and Mr. Brereton were thus agreed in the bold attempt to persuade the people of England that opium-smoking is not injurious. Sir Rutherford Alcock, though more careful in his language, sought, in his article in the *Nineteenth Century*, and also in his paper read at the Society of Arts, to minimize the evils resulting from the use of opium.

If these gentlemen could only prove that opium-smoking is not injurious, the very foundations of the movement now becoming so powerful for the suppression of the opium trade would be swept away; but unfortunately for the success of their enterprise, at the very moment when they were thus seeking to prove that opium-smoking 'is a harmless, if not an absolutely beneficial practice,' there were in England a number of men who, by their long residence in China, and personal contact with the people, and some of them by extensive travel in that country, were qualified to speak upon the effects of opium-smoking in China, with an authority, and a fulness of knowledge, compared with which the opinions of these apologists for opium-smoking were but as the small dust in the balance.

That an opportunity might be afforded these gentlemen to state 'the truth about opium-smoking,' it was resolved that meetings should be held in Exeter Hall, at which they should be invited to give the results of their experience. Nine of them (four of whom were medical men) accepted the invitation.

Mr. George Williams (*Treasurer of the Young Men's Christian Association*), Mr. James E. Mathieson (*Hon. Secretary of the English Presbyterian Missionary Society*), Mr. T. B. Smithies (*Editor of 'The British Workman'*), and Mr. T. A. Denny, united in an invitation to a large number of members of Parliament, and other persons of influence, to meet these gentlemen at a conversazione and conference preliminary to the public meeting.

The following pages contain the report of the proceedings, both at the conference and at the public meeting; and in view of the desperate efforts now being put forth to bolster up an infamous revenue, the testimony here given is of the utmost value.

On the one point, viz. the injurious effects of opium-smoking, the testimony will be found overwhelming. Let this be weighed in comparison with what has been said on the other side, and there can be no doubt what the conclusion will be.

Sir George Birdwood, Dr. Moore, and Mr. Brereton have each shown large faith in the credulity and ignorance of the British public. Never did the advocates of a losing cause display less wisdom in their methods of dealing with their opponents than did these gentlemen. Their utterances, to quote the words of a distinguished man, have been 'almost inconceivably foolish.'

Sir George Birdwood's letters have obtained for him a distinction which few of his professional brethren will envy. To say nothing of answers elsewhere, he is more than sufficiently answered in the following pages, and henceforth should speak tenderly of 'ignorant if well-meaning' persons.

Dr. Moore's method of justifying the opium trade is much more objectionable. Not content with attempting to show that 'opium is especially suited to the Chinese constitution, habits,' etc., he goes out of his way to paint the character of the Chinese in the blackest colours, and even to ridicule Christian missions to people in distant lands, with much more equally irrelevant. He has brought upon himself the well-deserved rebuke of the *Lancet*, which says:—

'Into Mr. Moore's diatribes against the exaggerated statements which have been made regarding the extent of the opium evil, and against a philanthropy which embraces distant parts of the world in its endeavours, we are not concerned to follow him. Exaggeration there has doubtless been, and needless exaggeration, for the facts are sufficiently conclusive without it. Nor is this the place for a discussion of the political and moral aspects of the Chinese opium trade. Mr. Moore's statements, which Sir George Birdwood anticipated "would furnish a complete vindication of the perfect morality of the revenue derived from the sale of opium to the Chinese," will seem to every unprejudiced reader to darken rather than vindicate the morality of the proceeding. The vindication consists of a violent tirade against the Chinese as the most drunken, debauched, and dissolute people on the face of the earth, and we are therefore justified in forcing upon them an additional intoxicant.'

A further extract from the *Lancet* is given in the Appendix.

Anything more ludicrous than Mr. Brereton's line of argument could not well be. The people of England were being misled 'by hearsay evidence,' 'and that of the worst and most unreliable kind.' He had beheld with concern the delusions now so common in England on the opium question, and he had come to dispel them, and he modestly entertained a confident hope that his efforts 'will prove in a humble way instrumental towards breaking up the anti-opium confederacy.' He had seen from afar the rising tide of public opinion, and he had come, Mrs. Partington like, with his mop to stem its progress! He had learned the truth about opium, and he desired to make it known.

But how had he learned 'the truth about opium'? Here is the secret in his own words:

'I have been the professional adviser of the opium farmer [who, he says, pays the Government of Hong-Kong £40,000 a year for the exclusive privilege of selling opium in the colony], and from him and his assistants I have had excellent opportunities of learning the truth about opium. I have thus been able to get behind the scenes, and so have had such opportunities of acquainting myself with the subject as few other Europeans have possessed. I knew the late opium farmer, whom I might call a personal friend, intimately from the time of my first arrival in China. . . . I knew him so intimately, and had so many professional dealings with him, irrespective of opium, that I had constant opportunities of becoming acquainted with all the mysteries of the prepared opium trade.'

What evidence could the British public get equal to that! He says that the conclusion to which his own personal experience has led him is, 'that opium-smoking, as practised by the Chinese, is perfectly innocuous;' and, wonderful to relate, he further says, 'I have never met any one whose experience differed from mine.'

It is almost needful to apologise for referring to the statements of Mr. Brereton at all, but he has published his views in a large book, which some, who have not lived at Hong-Kong, may quote as though it were an authority worthy of reliance.

Sir Rutherford Alcock is an opponent of a different type. It is to be regretted that, by his changed attitude, one who has done such good service in this question should now have to be classed with opponents. Mr. Fossett Lock, in his article in the *Contemporary Review*, has rather severely answered Sir Rutherford. Mr. Lock says that Sir Rutherford

> 'admits that, in a most important matter, which it has been his duty to study for years, he has been for years mistaken in his views, and misleading the public opinion of England. Now, upon fresh information, acquired since his duty to acquire it has ceased, he has completely changed his mind, and he appeals to the public opinion of England to follow him in his right-about-face movement.'

The Rev. F. Storrs Turner has also, in an excellent article in the *Nineteenth Century*, ably answered Sir Rutherford; but no better answer to Sir R. Alcock's recently expressed views can be made than that supplied by his own evidence before the House of Commons Committee on East India Finance in 1871. Until he gives better reasons than he has yet done for his new views, it will be felt that what he said so soon after his return from China is more reliable than anything he can say now.

That opium-smoking is injurious in a very high degree; that England did force opium upon China; that England now forces opium upon China; that the Chinese are sincere in their desire to put down opium-smoking; and that the native growth is no evidence of insincerity,—are facts most clearly shown by Sir Rutherford Alcock in his evidence, as the quotations given in the supplementary portion of this pamphlet will show. Other documentary evidence of high value to the same effect is also quoted.

Sir Alexander Arbuthnot has also written in defence of the opium trade. His article which appeared in the *Nineteenth Century* is moderate in its tone, and fair and courteous towards those who hold views opposed to his own; but like many other Indian officials, Sir Alexander allows the interests of India to fill the whole range of his vision. He says: 'It is sometimes forgotten that in the cry of justice to China, the duty of dealing justly by the people of India is apt to be overlooked.' The reverse of this is precisely the case, and in the cry of justice to the people of India, the duty of dealing justly by the people of China is apt to be overlooked.

Sir Alexander Arbuthnot, in showing the importance of the opium revenue, says: 'During the last twenty years the opium trade has supplied to the Indian treasury a net revenue of £134,500,000.' What if it has? The sum is immense, but if the source of the revenue is unsatisfactory, the amount cannot be pleaded in its justification.

If the people of England could but see for one hour the poverty and wretchedness, the ruin and death caused in China by the use of one million pounds worth of opium, they would be horrified. What must be the extent of the desolation caused in China by the use of opium enough to yield the Indian Government a net revenue of £134,500,000?

And yet Sir Alexander can dwell with complacency upon what this opium revenue has done for India! 'Without the opium revenue,' he says, 'the education of the natives of India could never have been attempted upon its present scale; the funds available for the administration of justice must have been largely curtailed; the cheap postage and the telegraph could not have been introduced; the police must have been left upon its old inefficient footing; the expenditure upon public works must have been very much less than it has been,' etc. One reads such words with inexpressible amazement.

Funds available for 'the administration of justice,' derived from a trade which, in its origin and in its continuance, has been one of the greatest acts of injustice the world has ever seen! How incongruous the thought! If 'the funds available for the administration of justice' in India have been obtained by the perpetration of injustice in China, what then? If the education of the natives in one country has caused the destruction of the natives in another, what then? If efficient police in India means the corruption of officials in China, what then? If cheap postage, telegraphs, public works and other improvements in India involve the deterioration of China, what then? Must we, with our eyes opened to see that these things are so, go on in our wrong-doing? Surely Sir Alexander Arbuthnot and other Indian officials would not, could not plead for the Indian opium revenue if they knew all that its maintenance involved in China.

The following pages will in some measure reveal this to them. Here are the testimonies of eye-witnesses, than whom none better qualified to speak on the subject can be found. They are all tried and trusted men, whose sincerity and truthfulness are above question. Put on one side the opinions of Sir George Birdwood and Dr. Moore (neither of whom ever set foot in China), and the statements of the solicitor from Hong Kong (who cannot speak the Chinese language), and on the other side put the personal experience of the eleven missionaries whose testimony these pages give, and whose united period of residence in China exceeds 150 years, and then let any one say whether there can be a moment's doubt which is most to be relied upon.

Testimony more worthy of confidence has never been given, and that it may be of service in helping to form public opinion at the present stage of the controversy it is now published, with other evidence of unquestionable authority. If it were merely to counteract the unwise utterances of some to whom reference has now been made, the collection of this evidence would not have been necessary; but when men like Major Baring in high authority, while generously acknowledging the high motives of those who are seeking the suppression of the opium trade, repeat and endorse some of the same erroneous views, it is needful to have at hand authoritative answers to their misleading statements. Let their assertions be carefully examined, and the whole subject investigated, and there can be no doubt what the result will be.

The new defenders of the opium trade profess to have come forward to instruct the public, but as Mr. Turner has well said, 'when the ignorance was denser than it is now, these learned experts were silent;' and he adds, 'One may be forgiven for surmising that it is not the ignorance, but the knowledge of the British public, which they dislike.' The excuses for the opium trade which one or other of its defenders have urged may be thus summarized:

1. That opium-smoking is not very injurious.
2. That the British Government has never forced opium upon the Chinese.
3. That the Chinese are not sincere in their professed desire to put down opium-smoking, and that the cultivation of the poppy in China is proof of their insincerity.

4. That if we do not send opium to China, others will.
5. That if the opium trade was forced upon China, we are not now responsible for what others did long ago.
6. That if opium is injurious in China, it is no worse than intoxicating drink in England.
7. That India cannot do without the revenue derived from the opium trade.

These excuses are all more or less fully dealt with in the following pages, but most of them have no relevance whatever to the one great question at issue.

As so many seem to have no clear apprehension of what this one question is, it may be well to state it once again.

It is, that England, by compelling the Government of China to admit into China a drug which is a source of impoverishment and ruin to the people, commits a great national injustice, and that we ought not any longer to continue this injustice, but to allow the Government of China liberty to admit or not to admit opium, as in the interests of the people of China it may deem best. Can anything be more reasonable?

This is the one great contention of those who are seeking the suppression of the opium trade. All other points are secondary, and of little importance compared with this.

Despite all that has been said, upon incontestable authority, as to the fearful evils resulting from the use of opium in China, we have unrighteously persisted in forcing it upon that unhappy country. This we have been doing for many years. Cardinal Manning, at the Mansion House meeting, said:—'It has been going on now for a period of forty years. By means that are secret, I mean smuggling; by means that are violent, I mean war; by means which I hardly like to characterize, which I will call diplomacy,—we have been forcing upon the Chinese population the consumption of a poisonous drug.'

This we have done, and have done notwithstanding the most earnest protests, the most touching appeals, the most humble entreaties of the Government of China. The distress of the Government, the sufferings and sorrows of the people, we have disregarded, and have relentlessly aimed at one thing, and that the securing a large revenue for the Indian Government, by the sale of our Indian opium.

More than sixty years ago Dr. Milne wrote:—

'The vast consumption of opium on this side of India is the source of so many evils to the people,—and yet of so much *gain* to the merchant,—that I utterly despair of saying anything on the subject which will not be treated with the most sovereign contempt. I cannot but regard it, however, as one of the many evils which hinder the moral improvement of China.'

And since then, many others of the noblest men who ever left the shores of England, have been almost heart-broken on account of the wrong done to China, and have done what they could to make our wrong-doing known; but the people of England have, up to the last few years, nearly all been deaf to their cries, and so the wrong-doing has gone on increasing in extent, until now the very magnitude of the evil, as represented by the immense revenue, is used as an argument for its continuance.

An examination of this opium question can hardly fail to leave the most profound and painful conviction that no right-minded man can study the character of our dealings with China in this matter of opium without being filled with shame and sorrow. The record, if faithfully written, will form one of the blackest chapters of history.

Having regard to the nature and extent of the evils consequent upon our dealings with China, it may be doubted whether any nation has ever more deeply injured another than England has injured China. And yet there are those who can point to the amount of the money gained by our unrighteousness, and the difficulty of doing without it, as though that condoned our sin.

What notion of the justice of Him who rules the world must he have, who supposes that we can commit such exceeding wickedness and yet escape retribution!

Mr. Henry Richard only expressed what thousands feel, when, at the close of his admirable speech on the opium question in the House of Commons in 1876, he said:—

> 'I am not ashamed to say that I am one of those who believe that there is a God who ruleth in the kingdom of men, and that it is not safe for a community, any more than an individual, recklessly and habitually to affront those great principles of truth, and justice, and humanity, on which, I believe, He governs the world. And we may be quite sure of this, that in spite of our pride of place and power, in spite of our vast possessions and enormous resources, in spite of our boasted force by land and sea, if we come into conflict with that Power, we shall be crushed like an eggshell against the granite rock.'

This view of the matter is left out of account by those who consider the opium revenue so much clear gain. There is ample reason for believing that though what is called the 'net revenue' derived by the Indian Government from opium during the last forty years has exceeded £200,000,000, the real net money gain to India has not equalled a single sixpence. On this point we invite attention to the views expressed by Sir Arthur Cotton, Cardinal Manning, and others, which will be found pp. 95, 96.

That the difficulties in dealing with the matter are now exceedingly great none can deny. A course of wrong-doing cannot be long followed by a nation, any more than by an individual, without the difficulty of reverting to a right course being immensely increased.

The statesman who breaks the bonds of his official surroundings, and, Indian officials notwithstanding, resolves in this matter of opium to do justice to China, will need to be a strong man; but he will need to be a much stronger man who will successfully resist the efforts of those who are resolved never to rest until our national complicity in this iniquitous business is brought to an end.

He who is resolved that the opium revenue shall be maintained, and that the Chinese Government shall not be free to admit or not to admit our Indian opium, must take it into account that he has the Christianity of England to fight, for the conscience of England is now awaking.

The Friend of India thinks it 'hard to believe that any moral scruple could in the scale weigh down seven millions sterling a year, that the indulgence of any sentiment could be purchased at such a price.' But when 'sentiment' is only another word for a firm and conscientious conviction of what is right and just, it is a power that can do strange things.

It must, however, be remembered, that while those who seek the suppression of the opium trade demand first and chiefly that China shall be free to admit or not to admit opium, there are other considerations which, though subordinate, are of very great importance.

They consider it no small thing that the commerce of England should be sacrificed for the sake of the opium revenue. That it has been, the facts of the case plainly show. But for the opium trade China would have been long ago a market of vastly more value to British manufacturers and merchants than it has yet become. The following figures are significant:—

The export of opium from India to China for the year 1880-81 amounted in value to £10,244,442.

The exports from the United Kingdom to China, including Hong-Kong and Macao, were—

Cotton yarn and cotton,	£6,178,344
Woollens,	£1,279,620
Metals and sundries,	£2,024,858
	£9,482,822

This is the amount of our exports to a country containing a population numbering hundreds of millions. If manufacturers and merchants will study the opium question in its bearing on the interests of British commerce, they will marvel at some of the lessons to be learned. (See 'Opium Trade and British Commerce,' p. 73.)

Another important consideration is, that it is no light thing that a line of conduct should be followed by England which, instead of securing the goodwill of the Chinese, is having a contrary effect, and is causing towards England a deep distrust and dislike. The goodwill of the Chinese, whose power and influence in the East are rapidly increasing, would be to England a source of strength, as their ill-will may become a source of no small danger. Our opium policy in this respect is the very opposite of all that wise statesmanship would dictate.

Moral, commercial, and political considerations, it will thus be seen, all combine to prove the importance of suppressing the opium trade.

A further consideration must be mentioned. It is, that Indian interests are imperilled, and serious financial derangement risked, by a continued dependence upon a source of revenue so precarious as the opium revenue is admitted to be.

The opium revenue is in danger; its own friends say so. They consider it in danger from the extensive growth of the poppy in China. The danger from this source we consider too remote to cause any immediate apprehension. In face of the fact that, with an increasing cultivation of the poppy in China, the Indian opium revenue has continued to increase, and that the limit of the power of consumption in China has not yet been reached, there is not much reason to expect that, beyond a possible disturbance in price, the Indian opium revenue will be seriously diminished by the native growth for some time yet.

There is, however, danger from other sources. The Chinese Government, chafing under a sense of long-continued injury, may settle the matter by a word. If to-morrow morning the Government of China informed Sir Thomas Wade, Her Majesty's representative in China, that on and after January the 1st, 1883, the Government of China would not admit opium any longer, what would be the result? There would be some vapouring about 'Violation of treaty rights,' 'The power of England defied,' 'Insult to the British flag,' and the usual appeals to popular ignorance; but would any Government in this country venture to go to war again to force opium upon China? Would public opinion allow such a course? There is reason to believe that it would not. What, then, would be the fate of the Indian opium revenue? It would be cut off at a stroke. If, however, it should happen that evil counsels prevailed, and that, in spite of the moral feeling of the country, we were dragged into war, it would be a war very different from the China wars of former times. We may not doubt on which side victory would ultimately lie, but the cost in blood and treasure would be unexampled, for China during the last twenty years has made extraordinary progress in the development of her defensive resources.

How near we may be to some such resolve on the part of China not to admit our opium any longer, we do not know; but there is good reason for believing that some of the most influential men in China are only waiting the time when, feeling strong enough to risk the consequences, they may announce their determination not to submit any longer to that clause in the Treaty of Tientsin which, to the incalculable injury of their country, compels them to admit opium. Such an ending of our opium trade would be ignominious, and would fix upon this country the indelible stain of having held to the trade as long as it could. Nor would this be all; our future relations with China would be damaged for generations to come.

The most certain danger to the Indian opium revenue may, however, be looked for where it certainly ought to be found, viz. in the action of the people of England. It is shameful that this action has been so long delayed; but the country is now becoming aware of the wrong that has been done in its name, and has commenced a movement, which is rapidly gathering force, and which will undoubtedly bring England's connection with the trade to an end.

The Friend of India and Statesman, alarmed at the prospect of the opium revenue being lost, says: '*If a certain number of electors joined the movement, so as to make it worth a hundred votes or so to each candidate at a Parliamentary election, the thing would be done.*' This is undoubtedly true; but the same authority cherishes the delusion that if the opium monopoly were abolished, the revenue might be saved. The article is altogether most remarkable. Much of it is given in the Appendix, pp. 87, 88, and will amply repay a careful reading.

Major Baring in his Budget speech discussed this question with great fairness and ability, and clearly showed that if the opium revenue is to be maintained, the monopoly cannot wisely be abolished. One important consideration he did not name, though it might have been present to his mind, viz. the improbability of private capitalists risking enormous sums of money by ventures in connection with a trade the continuance of which they could not safely count upon for a single year.

The abolition of the monopoly in order to get rid of the odium attaching to it, and in order that the revenue may be the more permanently secured in another form, would be little less than an attempt to deceive the people of England, and would not touch the morality of the question.

While respectful towards opponents, Major Baring unhappily appears to be driven by the exigencies of his position to defend the trade. He avoids the folly of those who assert the non-injurious effects of opium-smoking, but on the most important point he takes a false position, and contends that opium is not forced upon China. The evidence in the supplementary portion of this publication will have been selected to little purpose if Major Baring's error on this important point is not abundantly proved.

A further proof, if further proof were needed, is afforded by the terms of the notice of motion in the order-book of the House of Commons. All that Sir J. W. Pease asks for is that the Government of China may be free to act in the matter of opium as it may judge best. Why ask for freedom for China if China is free already? If China is not forced to admit opium, there is nothing to prevent the Government giving cordial assent to the motion. Will the Government do this? A vote on this motion, one way or the other, would be worth a good deal.

The *Friend of India*, though mistaken about the means whereby the revenue may be saved, has very clearly indicated where the power lies by which it can be ended, viz. 'in a certain number of electors,' and all that is needed to secure the action of the 'certain number of electors' is that they shall understand what it is we have done and are doing by our opium trade. This is the opinion of those best acquainted with the question.

Sir Edward Fry says:—

'I have such faith in the good feeling of my countrymen, that I believe that if they could once realize what it is that we have done and are doing as regards opium, they would rise as one man, and get rid of the accursed thing, which, as sure as there is a moral government in the world, will one day or the other find us out.'—*England, China, and Opium*, p. 6.

The Rev. Griffith John says:—

'Attempts were sometimes made to palliate the sin of the trader, and to make light of the evil effects of the drug. On both points our utterance must be clear and emphatic. We *know* that opium is a *curse* —a curse *physically*, a curse *morally*, and a curse *socially* to the Chinese, and this fact we must declare in loud, ringing tones. . . . It is our duty to appeal to the great heart of England—for she has a heart, and when that heart begins to beat warmly on the question, this foul blot on her escutcheon will soon be wiped off.'—*Speech in the Shanghai Conference*, 1877.

THE REV. DAVID HILL SAYS:—

'It had been said that this traffic produced a revenue to India of eleven million pounds sterling per annum. It mattered not whether it were eleven million or eleven hundred million; if the *source* of revenue be immoral, the *amount* of it cannot justify its collection. He thought the English public were not at all acquainted with the real state of the case, and that if it were plainly laid before them, we might hope to see the traffic suppressed.'—*Speech in the Shanghai Conference,* 1877.

Light is spreading, and this trade cannot live in the light. Three or four hundred missionaries scattered throughout China cannot live among the people without the truth about opium-smoking being known to them, and through them to all who are interested in their work.

There are also powerful agencies at work in England.

In the diffusion of information sorely needed, the Society for the Suppression of the Opium Trade has done a work which has given it a just claim to public gratitude and support.

Much, however, remains to be done, and the society now referred to should have a more widespread and generous support, and to this should be added the further aid of energetic personal effort on the part of every one who is convinced that it is an unrighteous thing to force an injurious drug upon China.

We owe much to China. We have deeply injured the people of that land. The evil we have done we cannot undo, and the evil now being done we cannot prevent. Multitudes, tempted by the drug we have supplied, and compelled their Government to admit, have formed habits which will be the ruin of their families and themselves. We have set in motion forces of evil which we cannot now control, and this we, as a people and nation, are responsible for. If it had been the action of individual Englishmen which had caused all the ruin and death which has been consequent upon the use of our opium in China, it would have been bad enough; but it has been through the action of the British Government that the evil has been wrought, and the sin of this rests upon us all. We are individually responsible.

Our national connection with the traffic must, at all costs, be ended. Thousands are resolved that it shall be, and are working to this end. What is needed to aid them in their work? Nothing so much as the unimpeachable testimony of those whose position and experience qualify them to speak upon the question with an authority none can gainsay. To supply such information the following pages have been published.

B. BROOMHALL.

2 PYRLAND ROAD, MILDMAY, N.,
May 1882.

THE TRUTH

ABOUT

OPIUM-SMOKING.

PROCEEDINGS AT A MEETING

HELD IN THE

COUNCIL ROOM, EXETER HALL, LONDON,

ON WEDNESDAY, MARCH 15, 1882.

THE CHAIR WAS TAKEN BY THE RIGHT HON. LORD POLWARTH.

THE meeting was opened with prayer by the Rev. H. GRATTAN GUINNESS.

The CHAIRMAN.—Gentlemen, the object of our meeting is not to make speeches upon the subject at this time, but to put direct questions, that those who are well acquainted with China may give us direct answers in as concise a form as possible, and distinctly state to us that which it is important for the public generally to know.

Certain statements have been made publicly with reference to the opium traffic. It is very important that those who have a thorough knowledge of China, and acquaintance with the Chinese people, and the bearing of this opium question upon them, should have an opportunity given them to state their opinions, and to give the facts as far as they have come under their cognizance, that the public generally may be enlightened upon this subject, and that views which have been put forward may be sifted and answered.

There is one question which I should like to introduce to the meeting. It has been said that opium-smoking is of itself absolutely harmless. Is that statement true? And what is the general effect on the opium-smoker mentally, physically, and morally? Perhaps some gentleman who has had acquaintance with China as a medical man will be able to answer that in the first instance. Perhaps Mr. Collins, who was twenty-three years in China, will be able to give us his opinion with reference to that question.

Rev. W. H. COLLINS, M.R.C.S.—I feel very little difficulty, indeed, in giving an answer to this question, and one most totally opposed to Sir George Birdwood. Sir George Birdwood most evidently is utterly ignorant of the subject on which he has written. He never could have written as he has, had he seen and known what I have seen and known.

The question is, What is the effect upon the Chinese mentally, physically, and morally? My experience is, that they suffer less mentally than in any other way; but they do suffer. The whole man suffers. But physically and morally they are most thoroughly deteriorated by opium-smoking. It destroys a man's energy for work. If he is a labourer, as many of them are, he must at a certain time go to his opium pipe. He cannot continuously labour as a healthy man does, but when the time for his pipe draws near, he is miserable and wretched until he can go and take it. Then he is restored for a time to apparently perfect possession of his faculties, because opium-smoking is not, as many imagine, only a soporific. It is a powerful stimulant, and when a man takes his pipe he is revived, and goes forth to his work again.

I have no doubt that all who have been in China have had experience with an opium-smoking teacher. As the time for his pipe draws near, he gets miserable. He begins to nod over his book; and if the time is prolonged, he will get thoroughly wretched until he can get away. We never would willingly get opium-smoking teachers, and therefore he conceals the real cause of his appearance, and goes away on some pretext, which, when he is dealing with one who is a novice in China, is very easy; and then he gets his pipe, and he comes back another man, and goes on with his work. But then you must remember that the interval between the pipes gradually shortens. At first he smokes probably twice a day, but a man must take more and more opium, as the months and years pass on, to keep up the required effect on his constitution. A man who is a labourer becomes a wreck in the course of a few years, utterly unfit for the work upon which his own livelihood and that of those around him depend. And then, as to the moral effect, every one in China knows what that is.

The Chinese are all of them more or less morally weak, as you would expect to find any heathen nation; but with the opium-smokers it is worse. The English merchants at Shanghai—those who introduced opium into China—would not tolerate an opium-smoking servant in their employ at the time I was living there, for he could not be depended upon. So it is with the Chinese themselves. They will not willingly do so. The smoker becomes morally weak. His selfishness becomes intense. One reason is, that he must supply his pipe at all hazards, and at all costs to those who are around him. The opium-smoker will steal anywhere and everywhere in order to supply his pipe, and nobody in any important business would in any way depend upon a man who smoked opium.

Opium is most generally smoked in China by the higher classes; and this is the great evil that it does to China, because the ruling classes are enfeebled by it, physically and morally, and therefore great wrong is done to the whole nation by the fact of the ruling classes being opium-smokers; and it may very well happen that even if England gives free leave to China to reject the drug they will not do it, because they have learnt to love it, and because they have in a great measure become dependent upon the income which is derived from the opium trade. Hence, unless a man were very strong-minded as a statesman, he would be unable to deal with this matter. You see we have incurred guilt in fixing upon the opium-smokers in China the love of the drug, and especially, as I have already said, upon the ruling classes, upon whom would depend the decision whether this drug should be rejected or not.

If there is any point which I can make clearer, I shall be very glad if questions are asked.

The CHAIRMAN.—Perhaps Dr. Gauld will say a few words. He has been a long time in China.

W. GAULD, M.D.—The question is still the general effect of opium, mentally, physically, and morally, upon the opium-smoker.

From an experience in hospital and dispensary work among the Chinese, ranging over sixteen or seventeen years, I can affirm, without any hesitation, that the statement of Sir George Birdwood is entirely wrong. There is no foundation for it in fact. He compares the opium-smoker with the tobacco-smoker. Now, in a company of Chinamen I could not possibly tell who was a tobacco-smoker and who was not; but if you put twenty Chinamen before me, and among them one man who has been long in the habit of smoking opium, I believe that I could point out that one man from among the twenty. That of itself is sufficient with regard to this comparison of tobacco-smoking and opium-smoking. You may ask how I could point out the opium-smoker, and the answer to this will be an answer to the question as to how opium affects a man physically. I can point him out by his appearance. The opium-smoker has a peculiar sallow skin, and, usually, blue, congested lips. This arises from the effect of the opium. It acts 'upon every nerve-cell, and probably every nerve-fibre.' At first the effect of it is slightly stimulant, but afterwards it is depressing and deadening, and the more a man smokes opium the more his whole system gets deadened. That is to say, his functions are not in a normally active state. This is manifested in a very simple way. For instance, the bowels of the opium-smoker do not act perhaps oftener than once in ten days, or once in fifteen days, and sometimes once in a month. I have known such cases.

It is the same with respiration. The blood gradually becomes less and less oxidized, and the venous system becomes congested. Hence you have that blue state of the lips and the shortness of breath of a confirmed opium-smoker. All these things show the effect on the body.

As to the mind, it acts through the brain, and you can easily see that the mind is affected by the effect on the brain. When a man takes opium, the immediate effect is stimulating, as we have heard from Mr. Collins; but that effect gradually passes off. His statement about the teachers I can confirm from my own experience. As a rule, these teachers soon get sleepy over their books. They cannot keep up their attention as ordinary men can. You may say, 'Why have opium-smoking teachers?' The reason is, that opium-smoking is so prevalent among the literary classes in China that we can scarcely get a teacher who is not an opium-smoker. This of itself shows the deadly effect that the habit is likely to have on the Chinese as a nation, because the rulers are taken from these literary classes.

Then, as we have heard, the man is affected morally. So long as he is a rich man, with plenty of money, not only to get opium, but also to get good food and clothing, the opium may not tell so seriously upon him or upon his family; but it must be remembered that the inevitable tendency of the opium-smoking is to gradually drain away the riches, and produce poverty; and as the man gets poorer, more and more relatively of his money goes for the opium, and less and less for other things. His family suffers, and at last, if he is reduced to poverty, he will not hesitate to sell his wife or his children in order to get opium. He will do without his food, if he has not money to procure both, and the last thing he will part with is his opium pipe.

Mr. E. B. UNDERHILL, LL.D.—The immoderate use of opium, there can be no question, produces the effect which has been spoken of, but I wish to ask whether there are a large number of men in China who use it moderately, and who are not carried on by temptation to use it immoderately; or whether it is universally the fact, that all who begin to use it, say in a moderate way, inevitably fall into its immoderate use? Is there a large number of men in China who use opium moderately, very much as men will drink moderately here, and not necessarily fall into a state of confirmed drunkenness?

Dr. GAULD.—I believe that there are many who at first do take the opium only occasionally, but I believe also, from what I have seen, that the tendency towards the habitual use of it is incomparably greater than the tendency to become a habitual user of alcohol. A man can take a little alcohol, such as a glass of wine occasionally at his dinner, without any one supposing that he is likely to become a drunkard on that account. At least many do it. But if a Chinaman takes opium oftener than a few times, such is the insidiousness of it, that in a short space of time he is all but certain to acquire the habit. And that is one point in which it is specially worse than alcohol. I believe that there are some things in which alcohol compares unfavourably with opium, as, for instance, with regard to the violence which is produced by alcohol; but with regard to the insidiousness and the tendency to become a habitual smoker, there is no comparison between opium and alcohol. Opium is far more seductive. That is the universal testimony, I believe, of those who have been in China.

Mr. HENRY VARLEY.—I should like to ask one question, my Lord. It seems from what we have heard that the ruling and literary men of China smoke opium very largely. Are we to infer that the lower classes are superior to the literary men in that respect, and that it is not a common thing amongst the poor?

Dr. GAULD.—A great many of the poor smoke opium. There are certain classes especially. For instance, the chair-bearers are almost universally opium-smokers.

Rev. W. H. COLLINS.—When we speak of the numbers who smoke opium, it must be remembered that probably not one per cent. of the whole population smoke, and therefore, if nearly all the literary classes smoke, there will be a very small number of smokers left in the lower classes. My experience has been chiefly in the north. Most of the gentlemen here represent the more southerly parts of China. My experience is that, amongst the labouring classes, comparatively few smoke; there are, in fact, scarcely any smokers in the agricultural districts. If in England the moderate drinkers and the drunkards together amounted to only one per cent., what should we hear of it? And yet what an outcry opium-smoking causes in China generally, though it does not involve more than one per cent. of the whole population!

Mr. HENRY VARLEY.—We have been accustomed to hear of the ravages of opium for the last fifteen or twenty years. I hardly know how to understand it. I do not know whether it strikes every gentleman in the same way. If it is only a question of one per cent., of course it is important to bring public opinion to bear against that; but we have been accustomed to think that it was a very widespread and ravaging curse; and I am afraid that if the thought gets out, it will appear that we have a very weak case.

J. MAXWELL, M.A., M.D.—My experience was almost wholly amongst the working-classes. To explain the difference between such statements as that of Mr. Collins and the experience noted by the other gentlemen who have just spoken, I may say that in the larger cities of South China one per cent. would not by any means cover the number of those who smoke opium; and in many cases 20 per cent. would not cover it, taking the adult male population as the basis of reckoning.

In the city of Tai-wan Fu, where the inhabitants are reckoned at something between 100,000 and 200,000, the Chinese estimate the number of smokers amongst the adult male population at something like one-half or one-third. I would not myself put it at that figure; but if we even put it at one-fifth or one-sixth, which is perhaps too low, you see at once how the statements about the ravages of opium-smoking are to be explained as compared with such a statement as that of Mr. Collins.

Then, again, if we take the city of Soo-chow, which is one of the largest cities in China, we have testimony which cannot be rebutted, that seven-tenths of the male adult population there use opium as opium-smokers. That explains how it is that there are places in China with regard to which you would speak of the terrible ravages of opium. On the other hand, I believe that the agricultural population do not use opium to any such extent as the population in the large cities.

My own experience would lead me to say that, physically, the effect of opium-smoking upon the working-classes is after a time quite manifest in the form of more or less emaciation. I do not believe that a working-man in China can smoke opium for any length of time without showing it in his flesh. He becomes emaciated. That is due simply to the general want of nutrition produced by opium. You will remark that fact amongst the working-classes far more manifestly than amongst the wealthy, well-to-do classes. The working-man is, perhaps, earning about 10d. or 1s. a day. He will have to spend about two-thirds of that to supply his craving for opium. One-third is left for the food. If any stress comes,—such as days of sickness, or failure of work, or anything of that kind,—he has necessarily to stint himself in his ordinary food. The consequence is, that the effect of the opium becomes much more rapidly manifest, and he is exposed in that way to the onset of disease, and of death from disease, in a way in which an ordinary working-man who is not an opium-smoker is not exposed. That is a point which must always be kept in view in connection with the working-classes. The effect is very much more quickly visible in them than it can possibly be in those who have plenty to eat and drink, and who are not necessarily deprived of food by want of work.

Then, as to the mental effect, I have no hesitation in saying that the effect upon the physical system is also more or less manifest in producing a certain dulness and lethargy of intellect amongst the opium-smokers. You cannot meet with a confirmed opium-smoker and speak with him without feeling that the man is not 'all there,' even mentally. He can answer your questions, but he has not the sustained mental vigour of the non-smoker. The testimony of the Chinese themselves is quite distinct—that the whole man is affected; that he is not only physically, but also mentally and morally affected.

And then as to the moral element, you have what I think no one can gainsay, and that is the testimony of the Chinese themselves. All through the South-Eastern provinces of China—I do not speak of Western China, I leave that altogether out of account—but in South-Eastern China the opium-smoker reckons himself to be morally criminal, and not only so, but the whole population also reckon him to be so; and in admitting people into the churches, we should not be permitted by the Chinese Christians to admit an opium-smoker. We should be regarded as doing an immoral thing ourselves, if we permitted an opium-smoker to be admitted into the church.

Mr. THEODORE FRY, M.P.—My Lord, in reference to some of the first remarks of Mr. Collins, I should like to ask him whether he thinks that if the supply of opium from our own territories were to cease, the Chinese would increase their home supply? I know that this is a question which does not affect the responsibility of this nation; but still it is a point upon which our opponents argue very strongly.

Rev. W. H. COLLINS.—I have not the least doubt that if the Indian opium were withdrawn, the Chinese would vigorously *attempt*, and to a certain extent carry out, the prohibitions, which have been very rigorous, against the planting of the native opium. But if they were to prohibit it effectually now, what would be the result? A much larger supply of Indian opium would flow into the country, and a much larger amount of silver would year by year be carried out.

That their will is to prohibit it, I have no doubt. Of course, I do not mean all of them; but Li Hung-chang, who is one of the greatest powers in China, is in earnest in the matter. Tso Chung-lang, who is also a most powerful man in China, is also in earnest; and if these two men, who are the most influential men in the empire, are sincere in the matter, they would be able to a great extent to prevent the planting of opium. They themselves do not smoke it.

The CHAIRMAN.—It is very important that we should know the general effect upon the population of China. Perhaps some gentleman who has travelled into the interior will tell us what the effect really is, and how far that effect is obvious to those who live in China.

The Rev. F. W. BALLER.—The effect on the population is obvious to all who travel in China. In every town and every place that I have been to throughout about two-thirds of the empire, you can see the result on the population in misery, and wretchedness, and poverty, and moral degradation.

In Western China I suppose that there would be fully 50 per cent. or more of the adult population who smoke opium; and in that part the population are the most miserable and wretched that you could meet with in any part of China. In proportion as the habit increases in different states, in that proportion do the population sink, and poverty and misery and all sorts of crime follow as the result. A man would need to be in China only a very little time before the evil effect of opium-smoking would be very apparent to him indeed.

Rev. J. SADLER.—I merely wish to say a word with regard to the spread of this evil. It ought to be remembered that in some parts of China, according to the testimony of the Chinese themselves, the opium shops are becoming as numerous as the rice shops.

Supposing only one man of a family be a smoker, the misery which he will cause will spread over his whole family. It may likewise spread over the family of his sons and others of his relatives, because the Chinese are accustomed to live very many under one roof, and they have one purse, and therefore the misery is simply incalculable, although only a few men should smoke. There is another thing to be looked at with regard to the spread of the misery.

Opium-smoking is a thing of comparatively recent date; and if it has grown already to such immense proportions, what will it do in the future, going on only at the rate at which it is spreading now? If these things are taken into account, it will be readily understood that the miseries are as great as ever they have been represented. I remember some years ago translating a ballad that the Chinese had themselves prepared, and which had very caustic remarks on the opium-smoker, bearing out exactly what Dr. Maxwell has said; and afterwards I read it to one or two Chinese friends, and everything which was there stated as to the abject misery of the opium-smoker was corroborated by them; and further, there was a most impressive allusion made to the utter ruin of the smoker himself, and then of his property, and then of the sale of his children and his wives, and even of himself in some cases; and therefore I think that we must be deeply impressed with the fact that what we have heard of the misery caused by opium-smoking is certainly true.

The CHAIRMAN.—Perhaps Dr. Galt, who has been a good while connected with China in medical work, will state his opinion about the first question that has been put.

J. GALT, M.R.C.S.E.—My Lord, I may just say a few words first about the number who smoke. Some years ago the Anti-Opium Society issued circulars to residents in China, asking for information on this question. Of course, it is a mere matter of opinion. There are no statistics. At that time I gave it as my opinion that 50 per cent. of the adult males smoked opium in the district with which I was acquainted. It must be borne in mind that the accounts we give are what we have seen in the part of the province or provinces we have been in. China is a very large country, more like a continent, and containing eighteen provinces, and when I say that 50 per cent. of the adult males are opium-smokers, I refer to Hang-chow, and part of the Cheh-kiang province. My opinion is that it is on the increase. And besides 50 per cent. of the adult males, a considerable proportion of the women also smoke. I noticed, when the returns were published, that the same proportion was given by a large number of the other gentlemen to whom circulars were sent.

I quite agree with what has been said already to-night about the action of the opium upon the smokers, that is, after it becomes a habit. They begin with a small quantity, it may be half a drachm, but the tendency is to increase. That quantity soon ceases to produce the desired effect, and in order to get the same amount of pleasant feeling and stimulant as at first, they have to go on increasing the quantity of opium until they arrive at an ounce or even more. I have frequently had opium-smokers coming into my hospital to be cured of the habit, not because they wanted to give it up entirely, but because they wanted to be able to commence again with a small quantity, and so get the same effect as from a larger quantity.

The results of opium-smoking are quite marked after a time. It produces a state of the body which is easily recognised—emaciation, and a peculiar sallowness of the skin, with dark teeth, and signs of indigestion.

My experience is that, although it keeps up the appetite, the action on the bowels is very marked. This is a thing that has been noticed in some of those letters in *The Times* lately, and an attempt has been made to defend the use of opium by saying that, because the smokers are in a great measure vegetarians, it does good by delaying the food in the alimentary canal, assimilating it, as it were, to that of graminivorous animals. That argument seems to me absurd. There is no analogy between the food of the two. That of the one is cooked and highly concentrated, is digested as quickly, and passes as speedily, into the system, as animal food does; whereas the food of graminivorous animals is largely composed of raw and gross matter, requiring long maceration and digestion.

I also agree with what has been said as to the mental effect of opium-smoking. It is a stimulant. For two or three hours the person goes on well, and does his work. When the stimulating action passes off, the man is weak and feeble, and wants to sleep, and unless he gets his dose renewed he is useless. I was talking this morning to a lady who told me that one day she had to wait for two hours in the burning sun while the coolies went and got their opium. That is a frequent experience.

Then as to its effect morally, they are slaves, and you all know what is the effect upon human nature of being slaves. They feel that they are degraded. There is a want of that independence, which is very useful amongst the Chinese as well as amongst ourselves, when one is free from any habit of that kind. They are looked down upon by their neighbours, and they feel themselves that they are degraded.

Dr. UNDERHILL.—I may ask Dr. Galt, as to those 50 per cent. who smoke, whether all are ruined by it in the manner which has been described, or what he thinks is the proportion of the 50 per cent. who ultimately fall into this degraded and wretched condition from the use of opium? I want to get at an apprehension of the extent of the evil and the mischief which it does.

Dr. GALT.—It depends a great deal upon the rank and social condition of the smoker. If the person is able to get good food along with the opium, it is a much longer time before the effect is produced; and, in fact, I believe that, with a good constitution, good food, nothing to worry them, and nothing to bring down their constitution, they may *occasionally* live to a good old age. The practice is of comparatively recent years, and it would be difficult to give an answer of any value. We see many people up to seventy or eighty, but I have not personally come across opium-smokers of that advanced age. In my district a very large proportion of the poor labouring classes smoked, and it took about three-quarters of their earnings. The average amount smoked is three drachms, costing perhaps 8d., leaving little for food; and as the craving for the opium is the stronger, it has to be satisfied first, until all the earnings go; and if the man has any patrimony, that too may go, and in very bad cases even the wife and children.

When a smoker falls ill with any serious disease, and is unable to smoke, he immediately dies, partly, it may be, from the illness, and partly because he cannot get his accustomed stimulant. The practice is for the friends to smoke and blow it into his face, that he may get a little of the effect.

Rev. W. H. COLLINS.—If I may answer that question, I certainly believe that nine-tenths of the smokers become morally and physically effete.

Sir THOMAS CHAMBERS.—What is the alternative, I should like to know? There is no nation in the world which does not take stimulants. What is the alternative in China to opium? Is it tobacco or any form of spirit? Because there is not a nation in existence that does not take stimulants. What would be the alternative, supposing that there was no opium?

Mr. DONALD MATHISON.—Before they commenced the smoking of opium during this century, they had tea, tobacco, and about as much spirits as they required. They had the opium pressed upon them, and, in fact, it was a great deal in that way that the supply created the demand; and we can show that. They would never have begun this system. It has swept like a scourge. It has increased from 5000 chests to 100,000 chests; and yet they have their tea and tobacco and spirits to consume as we have.[1]

Mr. WOOD.—I should like to say a word. I may be a little opposed to the general tone of those who have spoken, but I am sure that in spirit I am with them; and as I think that this meeting only wishes to know and to arrive at the truth, I trust that they will pardon me for just saying a word or two.

I think that a great deal of harm has been done in this cause, as in connection with intoxicating liquor, by intemperate advocacy. I have been four years in China, which appears a very short time after Mr. Collins and the others who have spoken; but as I have been engaged in commerce in that country, and none of the rest who have spoken have, perhaps I may be pardoned for occupying the time of the meeting. I was engaged by the largest house connected with this trade in China. It is the largest to-day, and it was so twenty years ago; and

---

[1] On this point, see Sir Rutherford Alcock's opinion, p. 82.

over two thousand chests passed through my hands during the last twelve months that I was in China at one port, and a very much larger business was doing at the other ports by our own people.

My own experiences of the effects of opium in the direction in which it has been spoken of are these: that there are thousands of Chinamen who take this drug moderately,—(A voice: 'Where?'),—just the same as our own people take a glass of wine or a glass of beer. (A voice: 'Where, please?') I am speaking of Foo-chow.

Rev. W. H. COLLINS.—Can they omit the pipe as we can leave off the glass of beer as we like?

Mr. WOOD.—Well, I do not say, I am merely making the statement. I do not say that a man can leave off his glass of beer.

Rev. W. H. COLLINS.—Oh, but he can.

Mr. WOOD.—But there are some that can not. Excuse me. If you will bear with me, there are many who take it in this manner, just as a man takes a glass of beer or a glass of wine. He may take two or three glasses of wine, but I mean without making a beast of himself. There are others who are more addicted to the vice. They take it more frequently. There are others, again, who find themselves entirely nerveless unless they take this stimulant, and they never enter upon making a bargain with any one until they have had a pipe of opium. There are others, again, who are lower down still, and to whom it is an absolute necessity before they can do anything. They are aptly represented by men among ourselves, who get up in the morning feverish and excited, having had no night's rest, being haunted with nightmare and so on; and it is impossible for those men to commence the day's business without a stimulating dram. I do not say that opium-smoking is not bad. I do not say that I should take part in it were I sent to China again. My business is now different entirely; but in the ordinary course I had to conduct this business the same as cotton business and sugar business and everything else.

I do not think that there is a gentleman in this room that takes his glass of wine, that can set his hand or his seal in opposition to opium. ('Oh, oh!') Is there any gentleman who takes a glass of wine in this room? There are doubtless; and I maintain that my experience entirely agrees with Sir Rutherford Alcock's, and that is, that you would see in one day in London twenty times the misery arising from intoxicating liquor.

The Rev. J. McCARTHY.—Will you kindly tell us whether you were able to communicate with the Chinese?

Mr. WOOD.—No.

The Rev. J. McCARTHY.—Will you kindly tell us how you got your information?

Mr. WOOD.—Experience.

The Rev. J. McCARTHY.—What experience?

Mr. WOOD.—Experience as a commercial man.

The Rev. J. McCARTHY.—With whom? With your compradore?

Mr. WOOD.—With many English. We had a smoking divan in our own place; and I could judge as well as I can of the evil as to the liquor traffic in this country.

The Rev. J. McCARTHY.—That there are thousands of men who smoke moderately?

Mr. WOOD.—Yes, and they do their work. I mean to say that the evil effects of the opium in China, as far as I know from books and from my own observation, are not comparatively great.

A GENTLEMAN. — Would you kindly allow me to say that the differences that we have had mentioned to-night range between one per cent. of the population and 50 per cent. ?

Rev. W. H. COLLINS.—Excuse me. Nobody has spoken of 50 per cent. of the population, but 50 per cent. of the male adults. The male adults are one-fifth of the whole. Half of that is 10 per cent. That is the utmost in the cities ; and in the agricultural districts very few indeed smoke ; so that, taking the whole together, it is not more than one per cent., which means four millions of men who bring to grief and destitution many millions of people.

The CHAIRMAN.—There is a question which I am not sorry at all that the gentleman who has just spoken has referred to—the question of drink. There is a question that I should like to get answered by those missionaries who have travelled a good deal in China, and lived there a good long time. Can you compare the drinking habits of England to opium-smoking in China; or do you agree with Sir Thomas Wade's opinion, which is as follows :—Sir Thomas Wade, in a memorandum of the revision of the Treaty of Tientsin writes thus :—

'It is to me vain to think otherwise of the use of the drug in China, than as of a habit many times more pernicious, nationally speaking, than the gin and whisky drinking which we deplore at home. It takes possession more insidiously, and keeps its hold to the full as tenaciously. I know no case of radical cure. It has ensured, in every case within my knowledge, the steady descent, moral and physical, of the smoker, and it is so far a greater mischief than drink that it does not, by external evidence of its effects, expose its victim to the loss of repute, which is the penalty of habitual drunkenness.'

I may say, from what I have heard to-night, that a good deal of what has been described gives one the impression that its effects are not very different from the effects of strong drink in this country. I should like very much to put the question whether, in the opinion of those who have travelled there and seen a great deal, and lived in the country, it is more insidious in its effects than strong drink,—whether it is more widely spread, and whether its effects generally are worse than those of strong drink or not ? Those of strong drink, mind you, I think are bad enough.

The Rev. J. McCARTHY.— I believe that the effect is very much worse. I believe that Sir Thomas Wade is able to speak with authority on this subject, because he is a Chinese scholar. He is able to hold intercourse with the people in a way that Sir Rutherford Alcock, long as he has been in China, is not able to do, or indeed few gentlemen who confine themselves to business transactions in China. I have lived twelve years in China, and I have been able to travel across the country from Shanghai into Burmah. During this journey, I met with people of all classes and of every condition; and from my continual intercourse and conversation with the Chinese, I have come to the conclusion that, bad as are the drinking habits of this country,—and I would paint them black enough if the time came to talk about them,—yet the opium-smoking of China is a great deal worse. It is a great deal worse, because it is an undeniable fact that, while thousands of men, and women too, use intoxicating drinks moderately in this country, the percentage of those who begin to smoke opium systematically, and continue moderate smokers, is so small that practically we may say that it does not exist.

The CHAIRMAN.—Can any other gentleman give us testimony on this point?

The Rev. A. E. MOULE.—My Lord, I have not been a medical missionary in China, but I have been there a good many years. It always seems to me, as to the question of the comparison between alcohol and opium, that there is no comparison whatever between the two. I think that we in England can judge of the effects of alcohol; and I really do think that the testimony of the Chinese should be taken on the question of opium. Gentlemen in this room who take a glass of wine do not feel pricked in their consciences in doing so. To take a glass of wine or beer is not a vice. But as to opium-smoking, I am perfectly certain of this—that in the opinion, I believe, of the opium-smokers themselves, or at all events in the opinion of every respectable and moral person in China whose opinion is worth listening to, it is a vice, and nothing but a vice, to touch the opium pipe at all, whether in moderation or excess; and therefore I cannot think that there is any comparison at all between opium-smoking and the use of alcohol in England. With reference to what Mr. Wood most truly mentioned just now, and what Sir Rutherford Alcock mentioned also, namely, the visible and brutalizing effects of the two, undoubtedly the palm of excellence as to non-brutality must be given to opium; and all shame to England be it that the crime of drunkenness is more outwardly abominable and more brutalizing than the crime of opium-smoking; only, as Sir Rutherford Alcock most fairly stated, and as Sir Thomas Wade has stated, and as those who have given reliable evidence on this subject have stated, intoxication is the exception, thank God, in the case of alcohol, but it is the rule and the object in opium-smoking, and therefore surely there is no comparison between the two.

One word more. With reference to statistics, I think Dr. Galt stated just now that we have no statistics as to the number of opium shops and opium-smokers. While I was living at Ningpo, I endeavoured to collect statistics, and I employed the native policemen, who, I fancy, are tolerably reliable persons. The opium shops are all marked by a well-known mark; and they reported to me, after carefully traversing the city, that there were 1700 opium dens in the city of Ningpo. Now, we know that drunkenness prevails to an awful extent in this great city of London, but there are only 10,500 licensed houses, including hotels and restaurants, in London with four millions of people. If opium shops existed in London in the same proportion as at Ningpo, there would be 17,000 of them in this metropolis. Is not that something perfectly terrific to think of?

I hope that the statements which have been made this evening will not be considered antagonistic, for they are not. The practice prevails to an awful extent. While I was in China I was informed by those who had reason to be correctly informed, that it was supposed that something like ninety per cent. of the Chinese army smoked opium; so I should imagine that one per cent. is as low as you can possibly put it if spread over the whole empire. At the same time, in many of the large cities the percentage is infinitely greater.

A GENTLEMAN.—That is the whole population of men, women, and children?

The Rev. A. E. MOULE.—Yes.

Mr. GEORGE WILLIAMS.—Many gentlemen, perhaps, in this room smoke, and they feel no guilt from smoking. They do not feel that they sin. I would like to ask Dr. Maxwell wherein the guilt of smoking opium differs from the guilt of smoking tobacco. Why is it a wrong thing to smoke opium and not wrong to smoke tobacco?

Dr. MAXWELL.—Because smoking tobacco is controllable, and does not result in utter moral ruin. The lust for the opium becomes so extreme that he must submit to it under all circumstances. No one who smokes tobacco is such a slave to it, that he must, under any circumstances, worship his tobacco. He must worship his opium.

Mr. T. A. DENNY.—I think my friend Mr. Williams does not smoke any tobacco. I should like to ask some authority in this room whether it happens often or happens ever, that men who have gone in for opium-smoking become reclaimed and give it up? With regard to alcoholic drinking, I think that some of us in this room could point to tens and hundreds of instances in England where men who have gone very far as drunkards, and who have been drunk almost day after day for years, and night after night, have been thoroughly and entirely reclaimed from drink.

Rev. W. H. COLLINS.—If I may answer that question, I will intrude again upon the meeting for a few moments. There is a great difference between the two countries. I believe that very few drunkards ever give up the vice unless the grace of God intervenes. I know of one case of a man who largely smoked opium who entirely recovered; and in that case it was the grace of God that did it. Of course, I assisted him in the way of medicines. There were two or three others whom I helped. I heard that they had given it up, but I could not bear witness that they had, for I never saw them again. But to this one man I can bear witness. But nothing can possibly be harder to abandon than the habit of opium-smoking. The habit of drinking cannot compare with it, difficult though it be to reclaim a confirmed drunkard.

Mr. CLARK.—I would like to say, my Lord, that I was connected with a mission in America amongst the Chinese, and I have known of two cases personally where, by the grace of God, the opium-smokers had entirely given up smoking the opium; so that I can testify personally to the fact that it can be done, though it is a very very hard thing to get it done. This is the hardest thing to overcome in the Chinese mission in America; that is the hardest work that they can find to do. Those are the only two cases that I have met with in my experience amongst the Chinese. I thought that perhaps you might like to know of those two cases, and know from one who has seen.

Dr. GALT.—My Lord, when I was in China my work was chiefly amongst opium-smokers, with a view to reclaiming them, and at that time about two hundred persons per annum gave up the smoking while they were in the hospital. What percentage returned to their habit I cannot say, but I have seen many of them years after they had left the hospital, and for anything that I could see, they still continued to be non-smokers. Giving up the opium is something dreadful. No one who has not seen it can form any idea. The stomach sometimes rejects everything, even a drop of water. They toss about in their beds, and they are sleepless for nearly a week. In fact, they are in the most abject misery it is conceivable for a human being to be in. That in a short time passes off, and they know that it will, and they come in hundreds every year to the hospital, and are willing to undergo all this misery that they may give up the use of the drug. They wish to do it, and they want our help; and yet the craving is so strong that they come only in small numbers.

(*The audience then adjourned to a public meeting in the Lower Hall.*)

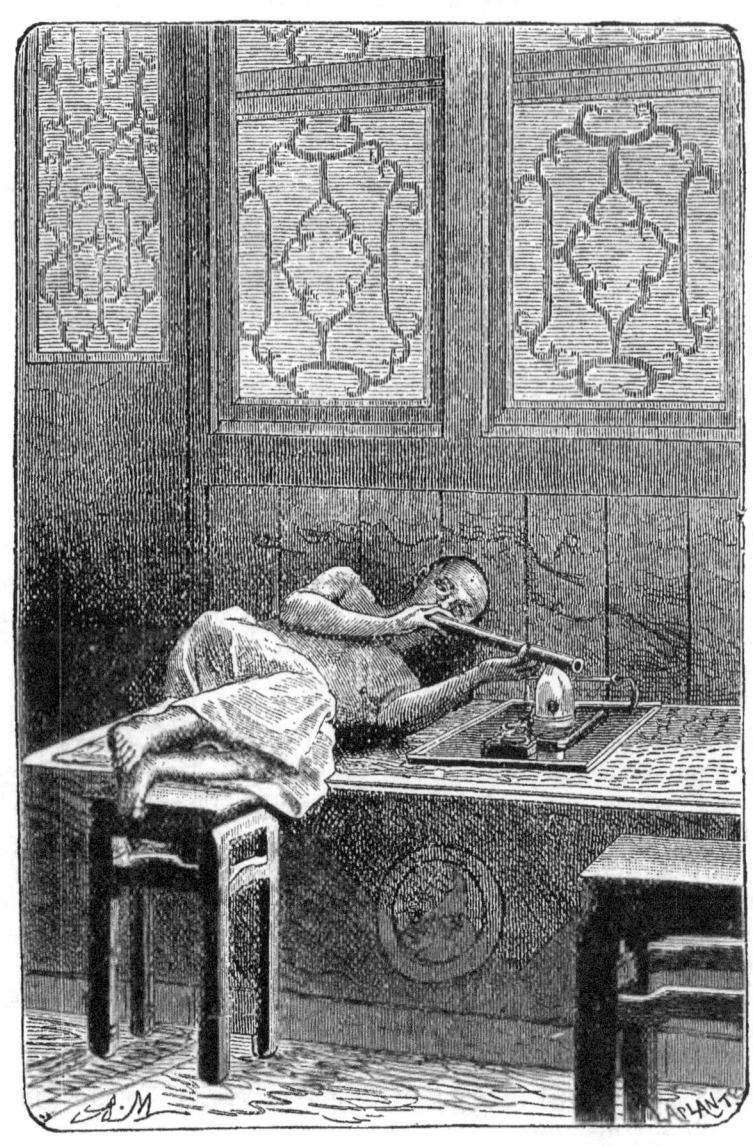

AN OPIUM-SMOKER.

PROCEEDINGS AT A PUBLIC MEETING

HELD AT

EXETER HALL,

ON WEDNESDAY EVENING, MARCH 15, 1882.

THE RIGHT HON. LORD POLWARTH IN THE CHAIR.

Prayer was offered by the Rev. DENHAM SMITH.

The CHAIRMAN.—Ladies and Gentlemen, Christian friends, I trust that I may be excused from saying much at the commencement of this meeting. I feel that it becomes me far more to be a listener. I am chiefly anxious that as much time as possible should be given to those whose experience and knowledge of China is such as to justify their speaking upon this subject. I shall therefore reserve any remarks I may have to make to the end, that as much time as possible may be given to those gentlemen who speak to you.

Mr. B. BROOMHALL (Secretary of the China Inland Mission) read a list of the names of gentlemen from whom had been received letters expressing regret at inability to be present.

THE REV. DAVID HILL,

Of the Wesleyan Missionary Society, sixteen years a missionary in China.

My Lord,—I take it that the announcement which has been given with regard to this meeting is of the utmost importance; that is, that we learn the truth with regard to the opium question. The dangers of exaggeration have been made manifest both on the part of the apologists of the traffic, and on the part of the opponents of it. I have in my hand a paper recently received from China, published in Shanghai under date January 31st. I find that the editor, who, I believe, is no friend to the Anti-Opium Society,—at least I think that I may say so,—gives his opinion with regard to Sir George Birdwood's deliverance on the subject; and I may be allowed, in the first instance, to read from this paper what is the opinion of the editor of the chief English paper in China with regard to this matter. He says:

'We have always taken what we believe to be a moderate view of the much vexed opium question, and hazarded an opinion that the evil effects of limited indulgence in the drug may have been rather overstated by philanthropists. But we confess ourselves somewhat staggered by the theory advanced by Sir George Birdwood in *The Times*, that opium-smoking is actually beneficial.'

He then quotes Sir George Birdwood's words : 'As regards opium-smoking, I can from experience testify that it is of itself absolutely harmless.' He also speaks of it as 'a perfectly innocuous indulgence,' and condemns the efforts of the Chinese Government to suppress it as 'despotic.' The editor himself then goes on to say:

'We regard this as rubbish of the purest type, and disbelieve it flatly. Nobody before, as far as we know, has ever ventured to deny the evil effects—moral and physical—of opium-smoking. The most that has been done is an attempt to show that it is not so prevalent a vice as it has been represented, and that the Chinese Government is less opposed to opium-smoking than to the opium trade. We have taken up this position ourselves on several occasions; but every man with his eyes open knows perfectly well, that among the Chinese at all events the results of opium-smoking are fatal and deadly, that the practice is condemned as on a par with the grossest sensuality by all Chinese moralists, and that no man feels the burden and agony of the opium despot more keenly than those who are in slavery to it. We do not mean to be flippant when we express an opinion that Sir George Birdwood would have been far better employed in twiddling his own thumbs than in writing such mischievous nonsense to a leading paper.'

The question is sometimes asked me, 'But is opium-smoking really as bad as it is represented?' Of course, that question requires definition and further explanation. I should require to know, in the first instance, how it has been represented, and then I should be able to give an answer to that question. I should like this evening to say a word or two, not so much with regard to the physical consequences of opium-smoking, although I will say, with regard to that, that during a sixteen years' residence in China, I can only recall one instance in which an opium-smoker said to me that he had been an opium-smoker for twenty or thirty years, and had experienced very little ill effect from it; but I have met scores—I may say hundreds—of cases in which the very opposite has been said. As to the moral consequences—and these, to my mind, are the most serious—they are universally deteriorating, so much so that the opium-smoker first of all loses self-respect, and then he loses the respect of his fellows.

OPIUM-SMOKING CONDEMNED BY THE CHINESE.

Opium-smoking in China is condemned by the public conscience. The missionaries throughout the whole country could not take a more direct course to ruin the interests of Christianity in that country than that of admitting opium-smokers into the Christian Church. With regard to the testimony of the Chinese themselves, I should like to bring before you this evening a few witnesses as to this matter. I may point you to the Government proclamations on the one hand, and to the religious tracts on the other, both of which class opium-smoking with gambling and licentiousness. It was not very long ago that in the town of Sheffield I had the pleasure of meeting with a Chinese gentleman who is in the employ of the Chinese Government, and, strange to say, whilst I was spending a very pleasant afternoon with him, a newspaper was brought into the house containing the report of the paper which was read by Sir Rutherford Alcock before the Society of Arts some few months ago.

This led to a conversation, in the course of which this Chinese gentleman told me that in the foreign legations of the Chinese Government now established in London, in Paris, in Berlin, in Madrid, and in Washington, there is not a single opium-smoker in the employ of the Government, and that the Chinese Government would not send a single opium-smoker to be engaged in any of the embassies abroad. One man did offer, but as soon as it was found out that he was an opium-smoker, his name was erased at once. He told me, moreover, that whilst he was engaged in the Foo-chow arsenal a few years ago, there were four thousand men in the employ of the Chinese Government in connection with that arsenal,—that over these men the Chinese authorities have a more direct surveillance than they have in other arsenals in the country, and that not a single man of the four thousand was allowed to smoke opium. If a man applied for employment in that arsenal, the question is asked him, 'Do you smoke opium?' If he answers 'Yes,' he is rejected at once. If he should tell a lie, and be admitted into the arsenal, he would be expelled as soon as it was found out. This will give you some idea of what the Chinese Government itself thinks with regard to this matter.

THE CHINESE WISH TO SUPPRESS THE TRAFFIC.

We are frequently asked now-a-days whether the Chinese Government would take any action to suppress the opium traffic, supposing the British Government took action themselves. In this very paper, which I received only last Monday, I have very striking testimony with regard to this matter. It is given by the correspondent of the paper in Tientsin, and if I may be allowed, I will read some passages from this correspondent's very long deliverance with regard to the opium question. He says:

'At the present time, both Li and Tso' (the two leading statesmen in China, whose influence is most wide and potential throughout the country), 'along with some other high officials, seem to be in dead earnest in this matter, and something is sure, therefore, shortly to be done. The private and publicly expressed views of these celebrated statesmen are well known, and are believed to be perfectly sincere. Those who enjoy direct and social intercourse with the Viceroy Li—and they have the best means of judging—tell us so. Diplomatic courtesy perhaps demands that their views as expressed to British officials should be modified. It is well known that they express pretty strong views to the representatives of the United States, Germany, etc.'

He goes on further to speak of the negotiations with regard to the li-kin, and the duties to be levied upon opium.

'The present duty,' he says, 'at the ports is Tls. 30 per chest, and the li-kin, which varies from Tls. 20 or 30 at some ports to Tls. 80 or 90 at others, is calculated at Tls. 50 on an average, thus making the entire sum received by China or her officials Tls. 80 per chest. This contrasts very strangely with the amounts we derive from the Bengal and Bombay opium, not to speak of the manufacturers' profits out of the monopoly. Tso proposed to raise it to taels 150, but this demand has been lowered to Tls. 120. The British Minister is willing to sanction a rise of Tls. 10, making Tls. 90 in all. To this the Chinese object. It is not impossible the bargain may be struck at Tls. 100.'

Thus we have, on the one hand, one of the leading mandarins in China—a 'heathen Chinee'—endeavouring to raise the taxation of opium in order to the suppression of it in his own country. We have, on the other hand, the representative of a Christian government endeavouring to bring this taxation down, the result of which course we must all know. I might go on further to quote from this article, but the time will not allow.

THE UNANIMOUS TESTIMONY OF MISSIONARIES.

The verdict of the missionary body throughout China is unanimous as to this matter. Not one out of the 350 missionaries in China would admit a single opium-smoker into the Christian Church. Only the other day I received a letter from one of my brother missionaries, and he told me that, in a town recently occupied by the missionaries, 50 per cent. of the adult population are addicted to this habit of opium-smoking. Mind I am not speaking of the whole country now. This is a very serious fact for the missionary, because, at the first onset, it excludes 50 per cent. of the population from the Christian Church. Half the population of this city are thus self-excluded, or excluded by public opinion, or excluded by the voice of conscience,—whichever way you like to put it,—from the Christian Church. That is to my mind one of the most serious matters. Then arises the question, Are these 350 Christian missionaries in China capable of giving an opinion on the subject? Do they speak the language? Do they visit amongst the people? Do they know as much of the people as gentlemen living in the open ports, who cannot speak Chinese, and who very rarely are found in a Chinese city? I take it that 350 men giving a unanimous vote with regard to this matter ought to settle the question, and that their testimony cannot be compared, ought only to be contrasted, with the testimony of those who cannot speak Chinese, and who very rarely are ever in a Chinese city.

THE REV. ARTHUR E. MOULE, B.D.,

Of the Church Missionary Society, twenty-one years a missionary to China.

I am afraid that some of those present at this meeting may think this platform rather packed, and that the speakers on this subject are partisans. I should like to open my brief speech with just a word on that subject. There is no *prima facie* reason why missionaries should be partisans on this opium question.

I think that *The Lancet* newspaper was perhaps a little hard on Sir George Birdwood the other day—not quite so hard as the *North China Herald* in the extract we heard read just now. *The Lancet* thought that Sir George Birdwood's opinion was greatly invalidated by the fact that he formed that opinion whilst he was still a student at Edinburgh. Now, many people imagine that missionaries form their opinion about the opium trade before they go to China; but the difference between Sir George Birdwood and ourselves is just here: we have been to China, and Sir George Birdwood has not; and what we speak of is what we have seen, and what we have heard, and what we have tested.

Really, there is no reason why a British missionary should take pleasure in denouncing the action of his own well-loved country, as contrary to the principles of national morality. Why should he like to use strong words of that kind? Why, really, to come to the facts of the case, some of the noblest benefactors of Christian missions have been the largest opium merchants in China; and it is a well-known historical fact that the opium wars did open China, and did bring about, as one result, the official toleration of Christianity in China. Therefore there is really no reason why a missionary should go to China and make up his mind that he will denounce the opium traffic as a bad and immoral thing.

WHY MISSIONARIES DENOUNCE THE OPIUM TRAFFIC.

The fact is, that we are brought face to face with the evil, and as soon as we are able to go and speak to the people, that is the first thing brought forward against us. I have had it hundreds and hundreds of times thrown back at me, when preaching in the open air, or in our missionary chapels. Just at the very climax of a discourse, as you are warming to the subject, and desiring to bring home to the people the blessed message, you have the question constantly brought forward, 'Who brings the opium? Who sells the opium?' In our previous meeting to-night the question was raised, whether there was any comparison between opium-smoking in China and intoxication in England. The dreadful shame brought upon England by intoxication has sometimes seemed to me like a terrible dream. In an illustrated Chinese book representing the outer barbarians, as the Chinese call those from western nations, how is an Englishman represented? With a bottle in his hand. Well, I hope that we are ashamed of that. But then, what are we doing for China? We are helping the Chinese to be demoralized with opium. Not content with our own bottle, we encourage them to use their pipe. You see, therefore, that missionaries who mix amongst the people, and hear their ideas on this subject, cannot help being—I hope not immoderate or intemperate, but certainly warm on the subject, and anxious to seize on every opportunity to try to bring information to bear with regard to it.

This meeting, according to the circular which has been distributed, is, I think, for positive testimony; and so, instead of endeavouring to moralize on the subject, I will bring before you some positive testimony. I may state, then, as a positive fact, that no Chinaman who is an opium-smoker will defend the practice; though he will excuse himself for at first adopting it. I believe my medical friends here present can corroborate the statement, that a very large portion of the Chinese opium-smokers have taken to the practice, under injudicious native medical advice, during some illness in which they have been recommended to try a whiff of the opium pipe; and the habit has thus grown upon them. The Chinaman will defend the beginning of it, observe, but he will never defend the habit as a habit. The Bishop of Victoria stated at the Newcastle Congress that a Chinaman is always ashamed of his opium pipe.

Now, as to the statement of Sir George Birdwood, that opium-smoking is perfectly innocuous, and very much like tobacco-smoking. May I venture to reverse the picture? I heard the other day that it is quite possible to have *delirium tremens* from tobacco-smoking. During my residence in China the Chinese have often told me that they have known a few cases in which intoxication has followed from the immoderate drinking of tea. Now, I believe that Sir George Birdwood's statement as to the innocuousness of opium-smoking must be placed side by side with that of *delirium tremens* from tobacco-smoking and intoxication from tea. If, on account of those very rare exceptions, you admit that tobacco-smoking is a vice and that tea-drinking is a vice, then I will admit that opium-smoking is a *virtue;* but otherwise, not so.

THE CHINESE CONSIDER OPIUM-SMOKING A VICE.

The Chinese denounce opium-smoking as a vice, and nothing but a vice. That is the general sentiment of the Chinese, and I wish to prove it by two instances. Some few years ago, at one of our missionary stations, a young carpenter had a very dangerous whitlow on his hand, causing him excruciating pain. A catechist, whose name I will not mention, though I know the man intimately, said to the young carpenter, 'I understand that opium has a soothing effect. I think that it will relieve your pain.' So he took the young man into an opium den. The carpenter was rather afraid to touch the opium, and so, in order to encourage him to take this 'gentle stimulant,' as it is called, the catechist lay down and took a whiff of the pipe, and then the carpenter took some; and they went out. This was noticed and heard of by the native Christians connected with the church, and they immediately started 140 miles down the country to lay information before the missionary. The case was inquired into, and with the full assent of the whole church, and the full consent of the poor catechist himself, he was there and then suspended from his employment for six months. It was felt that the opium den was a dangerous and immoral place, and that, however excellent his motive might have been, he was guilty of a grave mistake in taking the young man in and going in himself. If a man were to go into a tobacconist's shop, or into a hotel or restaurant, in England, to get a little gentle stimulant because he was suffering pain, would any clergyman or minister dare for a moment to turn such a man out of employment for six months? Certainly not. And do you think that the missionary would have dared to suspend that catechist if he had not been perfectly certain that not only the moral sentiment of the Christians, but the moral sentiment of the whole city, heathen as well as Christian, was at his back?

One more case and I have done. Some few years ago I was walking over the country from one of our out-stations to the city of Ningpo. One of my companions, whose conversation beguiled the weariness of the way, was a well-educated and well-spoken Chinese gentleman. He talked about all kinds of subjects; and I told him my message—the gospel of the grace of God. Just as we drew near to the city of Ningpo, he pointed to its walls and said, 'Do you know what is ruining the rising generation in our city?' 'No,' I said. 'The white and the black,' was his reply. 'What do you mean by that?' said I. 'The white powdered faces of the harlots and the black opium.' Observe that statement. He set vice by the side of vice; and that, I believe, represents the true moral feeling of the respectable people in China—that opium-smoking, be it in moderation or be it in excess, is a vice and nothing less.

W. GAULD, ESQ., M.D.,

Of the Presbyterian Church of England, sixteen years medical missionary in China.

My Lord and Christian friends,—We have been hearing to-night of the action of missionaries in China with regard to the opium. In connection with that, I should like to read a short statement of what Sir George Birdwood has said on the subject of opium-smoking. He says:

> 'I am not approving the use of stimulants. I have long ceased to do so. I am only protesting that there is no more harm in smoking opium than in smoking tobacco in the form of the mildest cigarettes, and that its narcotic effect can be but infinitesimal, if indeed anything measurable, and I feel bound to publicly express these convictions, which can easily be put to the test of experiment.'

Sir George Birdwood seems to have had before his mind the fact that his statements were likely to be contested, and he seems to have gone on the principle, that it was just as well to be hanged for a sheep as a lamb. From the comparison which he makes, one would suppose that we had only to do with the question of opium-smoking. It happens, however, that in the part of the country with which I am acquainted, the Chinese, almost to a man, smoke tobacco. Many of them drink more or less of intoxicating liquors. They drink whisky made from rice and other grains. The missionaries in China have many tobacco-smokers in the Church, and they have some who take more or less of alcohol; but they never dream of taking any ecclesiastical action in the case of a tobacco-smoker; nor do they take such action in the case of a man who drinks Chinese whisky, unless he carries the drinking to excess. Why, then, is it that they make an exception in the case of opium? Simply for this reason—that, as you have heard, the missionaries and the Chinese themselves look upon opium-smoking as a vice.

The taking of opium, even in small quantities, is certain, as a rule, to lead to the habitual use of it, and to becoming a confirmed opium-smoker. The moment a man begins to take opium, our alarm is excited, and we feel that he has begun a course which, unless he stops at once, is almost certain to land him at last in moral, physical, and social ruin. That is the reason why no opium-smoker is admitted into the Church in China. To show, again, that there is no comparison between opium-smoking and the use of tobacco, as I stated at the previous meeting, you cannot tell by the face of a Chinaman whether he smokes tobacco or not, any more than you can tell by the face of an Englishman; but if you take a score of Chinese and put among them one confirmed opium-smoker, a man who has had any experience of the Chinese, and especially a medical man, can point him out at once from his very appearance. The sallow face, the bluish lips, and the whole aspect of the man at once mark him as using this poisonous drug.

Now, how does this opium act? At first it produces upon those who take it a pleasant effect, and a delicious sensation, which they enjoy; but very soon this pleasant stimulating feeling passes off, and it is succeeded by depression. To remove this, the dose is repeated, and so the practice goes on from day to day, from month to month, and from year to year, and the Chinaman takes the opium as regularly as his meals, twice a day, or it may be three times a day, or even oftener. The longer he uses it, the more he has to increase the quantity.

A SAD FACT ABOUT OPIUM-SMOKING.

One very sad fact about this opium-smoking is, that it affects the best classes in China as regards social position. It is, so to speak, draining the life-blood of the best families in the country. It is true that if a Chinaman has plenty of money, and can afford to get good food and good clothes, and to have leisure, he suffers apparently least from the effect of opium; but the very use of opium, which is an exceedingly expensive article, tends in itself greatly to produce poverty; and those who are opium-smokers become so demoralized by the use of the drug, that, rather than forego their opium, they will do anything. They will sell their wives, they will sell their children, they will sell everything they have; they will give up their food; but the last thing that they will part with is the opium pipe. The Chinese have a special term for those opium-smokers who have reached this stage. They call them 'opium ghosts,' or 'opium demons,' on account of their emaciated appearance. They are perfect wrecks of human beings.

AN EXAMPLE.

One instance is, I think, worth a hundred arguments in this matter. We are told by many that opium-smoking is not the evil thing which it is called. I remember a well-to-do Chinaman from a distant village who came to the hospital. He was one of the literary class,—a scholar among the Chinese,—and a confirmed opium-smoker. After being with us for some time, he expressed a desire to be freed from the use of opium. We attempted to cure him of the habit, but such hold had it got of him, that in the course of the treatment he was reduced to death's door; and to save his life after he had suffered great torment, we were obliged to let him have the opium pipe again. In proof of his deep sense of the misery which the opium had caused him and his family, as soon as he began to get a little strength after resuming the use of the opium, he begged me to try once again if I could cure him of the habit. I said to him, 'Graduate, we have tried already, and you were almost dead. We cannot venture it.' His reply will show what was thought of opium by a man who suffered from it. He said: 'Teacher, whether I live, or whether I die, I wish you to try to cure me of it. I take all the risk.' He had with him a grown-up son, who was listening to his words, so I said that, on that understanding, I would again make the attempt. We did so, and by exceedingly careful nursing, along with the use of remedies, but not without great suffering on his part, and a close run for his life, he recovered, I am thankful to say, and was able to do without his opium. This is only one case out of many which might be given, and which show what the sufferers themselves think of opium.

You have heard to-night what the Chinese as a nation think of it.

Now I will give you an instance which will show the connection in the Chinese mind between this opium traffic and the people of Great Britain.

ENGLISHMEN AND OPIUM.

On one occasion, just in front of my hospital in a busy Chinese street, where hundreds of people passed daily, there was a Chinaman busy making beautiful little figures with pastes of different colours. There were figures of Chinese warriors, of idols, and of different eminent worthies, and in the centre there was one figure which at once attracted my notice. What do you think it was? It was the figure of an Englishman. He had a tall hat, which is a peculiar thing to a Chinese, and in one hand he had an umbrella, for we are usually seen in China, at least in the summer-time, with umbrellas to protect us from the sun. In the other hand what had he? A ball of opium! And so the Englishman was represented before all these people, moving in a constant stream along that busy street, as the man who brought the opium to China.

So much does opium-smoking affect the highest classes, that among the literati we can scarcely get one to engage as a teacher who is not an opium-smoker.

Many of the highest mandarins indulge in this habit to a large extent. I remember once giving the chief mandarin of the region around Swatow, who ruled over a population of several millions, a little entertainment with the magic lantern, showing him some European views. He was able to sit for about an hour, but at the end of that time the craving for opium had come upon him, and he could sit no longer. He got up and betook himself to his opium pipe, thus showing what a slave he was to the habit. That man was originally an able mandarin, and during a difficult period in the history of our relations with that part of the country, he acted with great skill between Europeans and Chinese. He was lately suspended on account of incapacity, and I have little doubt that that incapacity was largely due to his excessive use of opium. Many such instances might be given.

OPIUM-SMOKING SPREADING.

I may mention that this opium-smoking is spreading to a most alarming extent in China. At one time, as we heard, it was looked upon as a vice. So it is still; but I am sorry to say that at Swatow, when I was there, it was becoming so prevalent that a Hong merchant was considered inhospitable if he did not lay down the opium pipe for his customer, and give him some whiffs of it, just as a man in this country would make a bargain over some intoxicating liquor. I was told before I left Swatow that there was more money taken by the opium shops than by the rice shops. You will know the value of this statement when I say that rice is the staple commodity of life to the Chinese of the south. Rice is what they live upon for the most part; and if more money is gathered in by the opium shops than by the rice shops, you can understand to what extent the Chinese there are using opium.[1]

---

[1] A patient from the country told us that in his village of about 600 adult males some 50 or 60 smoked opium, say 10 per cent. of the adult males of this agricultural population. Other villages are similarly debauched, though in many the habit is as yet less prevalent.

This will show that whatever we do ought to be done quickly. The evil is rapidly spreading. We are told that no change can be made; that the Indian Government cannot afford to make a change. What does this amount to? It is a question of right and wrong. Cannot the Indian Government afford to do right? 'The throne is established by righteousness,' that is the only durable foundation. If it rests on a pile of opium chests, it must eventually come to ruin.

J. GALT, ESQ., M.R.C.S.E.,

Formerly in charge of the Church Missionary Society's Opium Hospital, Hang-chow.

My Lord, Ladies and Gentlemen,—I base my remarks upon the experience of about seven years' working amongst this class of people, with a view to reclaiming them from the habit. During the greater part of that time, I systematically put a set of questions to every opium-smoker who entered the hospital, with a view to ascertain, as far as I could, the real effects of it upon the smoker. The answers to some of these questions I am unable to give to a mixed audience. It is a purely medical subject.

With regard to that letter of Sir George Birdwood, which has to be referred to so often (not on account, in our opinion, of any intrinsic value in it, but because it has had so much publicity, and because upon it was based a leader in *The Times*), in which he says that opium is perfectly harmless. I may say that opium, as nearly every one knows, is a very poisonous drug. It is a complex article, and its chief ingredient is called morphia. The proportion of morphia varies greatly in the different kinds. Good Smyrna or Turkey opium contains 10 or 12 per cent.; India opium about 6; and the Chinese opium much less. Sir George Birdwood goes on to say that he thinks that this morphia is nearly all changed or destroyed in the process of making the drug into a smoking material, namely, by making an extract from it. Now this extract is very like what we in this country make of opium, and is a material in daily use among physicians. Instead of destroying the opium, the process makes it about double the strength, so that the smoking extract is about equal to the raw opium of Turkey, containing 10 or 12 per cent. of morphia. Then Sir George Birdwood says that this is a non-volatile substance, and therefore it cannot be introduced into the system by smoking. To that we would say 'not proven,' for the effects of opium-smoking upon a man are identical in kind with the effects of introducing morphia into the system by any other means,—by swallowing it by the mouth or injecting it under the skin. No doubt, smoking is the least hurtful of any means by which a man could take opium. It is, however, a very expensive way, for it requires ten times the amount when smoked to give the effect which one part would give if swallowed; and the smokers, when they do not find time to smoke, usually eat one-tenth of the quantity which they would have smoked.

THE TIME CONSUMED IN OPIUM-SMOKING.

Then, again, it was stated in that letter that it was a thing that just passed away in a whiff, so that not much could be introduced into the system. Upon an average, a smoker smokes three drachms of this extract in a day, and occupies about an hour's time in smoking one drachm. The time consumed in smoking is a very important point socially. A workman on an average smokes three drachms in the day, one in the morning, one at noon, and another at night. There is one hour wasted in the morning, when he ought to have been at work; and another at noon. The evening hour we will say is his own. Employers therefore object very much to have opium-smokers on this account, let alone other reasons; and we find that very often when a man begins to smoke opium he loses his place, and this loss of employment is one means by which he descends in the social scale.

The effect of the habitual use of opium has been pointed out already. You must be prepared to hear a good deal of reiteration, because our opinions are very much the same. We have lived amongst the people and seen the effects, and this should strengthen our testimony, for we have come from all parts along the coast of China, several of us strangers to each other, and have all the same tale to tell. After the opium-smoker has got habituated to the practice, and smokes a fair quantity, he usually becomes lean and sallow, but not always. Those in a good social rank, and who can procure good food, and whose bodies are not worn down by work,—who have nothing to do, in fact, but enjoy themselves,—smoke opium for a tolerably long period without much apparent effect upon them. Still, *as a rule*, you find that opium-smokers get lean and sallow, because the practice produces derangement of the digestive system. The appetite seems to keep up, but other parts, which one cannot go on to explain at present, get very much out of order.

OPIUM AND AGUE.

Then, again, you hear it said sometimes that opium is a great prophylactic against ague, and that the smoking is very beneficial to people in the malarious districts. I tried to find out the truth of this, and had great difficulty in coming to any conclusion about it; but my opinion was, that it had not much power to prevent ague. No doubt, when once the paroxysm of the fever is on, taking a smoke of opium may mitigate the attack; but smoking did not seem to have the effect of preventing the attack. I have again and again had opium-smokers resorting to the hospital when suffering severely from ague, and who have at once been bettered by quinine. And this leads me to remark, that even if opium did have a marked benefit upon certain diseases, which we admit, that is no reason for its habitual use by the masses. It is a splendid medicine. It has been called 'the gift of God.' But it is poor food.

The habitual use of it has a very marked influence upon the increase of the population. I find that only one inhabitant was added to an opium-smoking family during eleven years. In fact, one hundred and fifty-four parents, of an average age of thirty-three years, had only one hundred and forty-six children born to them during eleven years.

You have heard how the practice deteriorates them socially. They are *slaves* to the habit, and this fact makes them feel that they are low, and has a very marked moral influence. They feel that they are looked down upon, and the feeling of this helps to make them sink lower and lower, and do actions which, perhaps, otherwise they would not have done. Taken altogether, my experience is that the use of opium amongst the Chinese is injuring the nation physically, socially, and morally.

The Rev. F. W. Baller,

Of the China Inland Mission, eight years a missionary in China.

My Lord, Christian Friends,—It gives me very great pleasure to add my testimony to that which has gone before, and to speak of what I have seen and heard in China. I went to China in 1873. Since that time I have travelled in the seaboard provinces of Cheh-kiang, Kiang-su, Shan-tung, and Chih-li, and I have seen opium-smoking and its effects in those provinces. I have also travelled in the more central provinces of Gan-hwuy, Ho-nan, Kiang-si, and Hu-peh. I have both resided and travelled in these provinces, and I have seen the effects of opium-smoking in them. I have also during these eight years travelled in the north and north-western provinces of Shan-si and Shen-si, and I have seen the effects of opium-smoking in them. In addition to that, I have travelled in the western provinces of Hu-nan, Kwei-chau, and Si-chuen, and I have seen the evil effects of opium-smoking in that part of China. In the course of both residence and travel, I have mixed with all classes of the population,—the artisans, the official class, the military, the boat population, the commercial class, and the agriculturists—men, women, and children of all classes. It has been my privilege to mix with them, and have daily intercourse with one or other of them; and I have also seen them in the course of these journeyings, and in the course of my residence, in all the different occupations and relations of life—at their work, at their leisure, engaged in their different pursuits, at home, and day by day going about their various avocations; and I can say that in every one of these places.

It is a curse for this reason. As you have already heard, it takes a great deal of money, and brings the smoker to poverty; so that wherever you find most opium-smoking, there you find the most poverty-stricken people. The increase of poverty leads men to the commission of crime, and wherever you find opium-smoking to a large extent, there you find a corresponding increase of crime. And then, not only so, but you find all round that the opium-smoker is deteriorated and sunk in an abyss of ruin, and he himself knows it.

PUBLIC OPINION IN CHINA ON OPIUM-SMOKING.

Reference has already been made to the public opinion of China on this subject. I know something of the public opinion of China in two-thirds of the empire, and it is unanimous as to the fact that opium-smoking is an undoubted curse. I have seen the Government opinion of China in two-thirds of the empire, in the form of proclamations posted here, there, and everywhere; and the Government opinion is that opium-smoking is an unmitigated curse. And could I take you to-night to the many homes that have been blighted and made desolate; could I take you to hear the cry of the orphan and the widow who have been made such by this curse; could I but take the masses of London—could I but take the whole of England, and those persons who speak most in favour of this traffic—to see the things that I have seen, and to hear the things that I have heard; could the wail of the widow and the orphan come into their ears, I am quite sure that their opinion, and the public opinion of this country, would change without any hesitation whatever, and we should feel that the question of a few millions of money was as nothing compared with the removal of this curse from an empire such as China.

OPIUM-SMOKERS UNABLE TO RESIST DISEASE.

What proof have we that opium-smoking brings a man down and renders him liable to disease? It was my privilege, in company with Mr. Hill, who has already spoken to you, and with others, to assist in distributing the money so generously contributed by the British public to the famine districts of China. I was in the province of Shan-si, and the native testimony is that those who first suffered, and on whom the famine had the greatest effect, were opium-smokers. They were carried off first, and the non-smokers were able to withstand longest the ravages of the famine. This speaks for itself. I believe that in these famine-smitten districts, or I should rather say countries,—for they are more like countries than districts,—millions of men were carried off simply from the fact that their whole constitution was undermined by this practice of opium-smoking.

OPIUM-SMOKING ON THE INCREASE.

Reference has already been made to the fact that this vice is spreading. Unfortunately it is so. It is spreading in the form of social custom, and in the province of Ho-nan, in some places where it was the practice when a stranger went in to give him a cup of tea, that is being replaced by the opium pipe. The same holds good in Western China, and in Kwei-chau; and in the city of Kwei-yang, the capital of the province, that habit is obtaining to a very large extent. I have never been in any other province where so much opium was consumed as in Kwei-chau; and I have never been in a province where the people were so inert and apathetic, and where you had so much difficulty in arousing the attention, or doing anything at all with them, as in that province where most of the opium was smoked.

There can be no doubt that men who have been in China, who speak with the people and who mix with the people daily, know that these things are so. What have we to gain by maintaining these things? Nothing; but we do feel that we should speak for those who have not the physical power to plead for themselves with cannon, with sword, with bayonet, and with those things with which we have in time past pleaded with China; and we intend, God helping us, to take up, and that continually, and wage to the bitter end, the warfare on behalf of the millions of China.

The Rev. W. H. Collins, M.R.C.S.,

Church Missionary Society, twenty-three years medical missionary in China.

This is not the first time, Christian friends, that I have had the privilege of denouncing the opium trade from this platform. I may say one word upon a point which has been already touched upon, and that is, that we missionaries are said to be prejudiced upon this matter. What does '*pre-judice*' mean? It literally means judging beforehand. It is judging without testimony. I say that we are *post*-judiced—that we judge after testimony, and that we have received that testimony year after year, *ad nauseam*, both through our eyes and in our ears and in our noses; the testimony is, that opium, as has already been said, is a monstrous evil to China.

Now, with regard to the number who smoke it, I wish it to be always clearly known that we do not mean to say that any large proportion of the population smoke opium. Of course, more do in the cities, and fewer in the agricultural regions; but I suppose that, on the whole, not more than one per cent. of the inhabitants of China smoke opium.[1] But then, remember, what does one per cent. mean? It means from three to four millions. And who are those? They are the heads of the families; they are the bread-winners in those families; and upon those three or four millions there are depending some twenty or thirty millions of others, who are impoverished, and brought to a state of utter destitution, by the opium pipe which is smoked in the family.

DIFFICULTY OF HELPING OPIUM-SMOKERS.

I have tried again and again to raise opium-smokers from the Slough of Despond in which they are, and it is almost impossible to do it. During the twenty-three years that I was in China, I knew but of one case in which an opium-smoker was really rescued from the vice into which he had fallen, and that was a case in which a man became a real and earnest Christian. In almost all other cases they failed.

The Chinese themselves are making efforts against the practice. In Canton there is a native anti-opium society; and in several parts of the country, but especially in Pekin, as I know personally, there was established by the natives there an anti-opium refuge. Into this refuge came the smokers from the country round in considerable numbers. They supplied themselves with food, and maintained themselves there while they were doctored, and numbers left the refuge

---

[1] The numbers of those who smoke Indian opium can be approximately estimated by the amount of the drug received in China, and judging thus, certainly not more than half per cent. can smoke; but with regard to the opium grown in China, no approximate amount can be stated; its consumption may be, and probably is, much more than that of the Indian drug.

Several speakers estimated the smokers as 50 per cent. of the adult male population, not, be it observed, 50 per cent. of the whole population. Now, the adult males are about 20 per cent. of the whole, therefore 50 per cent. of them means 10 per cent. of the whole; and this is no doubt a fair estimate of suburban populations, and is quite consistent with the statement that 1 per cent. of the whole population smoke.

cured of their smoking, though I believe very few remained cured, because the opium-smoker, as you have heard, is of all men the most morally weak. They are utterly unable to resist the constant temptation that is put before them when they have been cured and have gone abroad again amongst their fellow-men. Any who may have seen the hospital report of Dr. Dudgeon, in Pekin, may remember there the case of a prince who was a victim to opium. He smoked nearly two ounces a day, and also took a large quantity of wine. Sir George Birdwood said that the two stimulants would not do together. This prince not only smoked two ounces of opium, but he drank fifteen pints of champagne daily. Dr. Dudgeon went to him. It was not difficult to wean him from the wine. That was soon accomplished; and at last he was cured of the opium-smoking, and became another man. And he walked out to call upon his preserver. But some time after he went to visit an aristocratic acquaintance, and the pipe was offered to him. He took it, he smoked, and he died.

This vice interferes very much, as you have heard, with the work of missionaries in China, and our indignation is kindled against it very much on that account. We constantly meet it.

When I was in Shanghai, there was a boy who had passed from our school there, and we had great hope of his becoming a Christian assistant, but he took to opium-smoking, and then broke open my drawer and stole a quantity of money. He was captured and brought back again, and I tried to raise him again and again, but at last he died in a ditch, covered with sores; and this was all through opium.

In Pekin, the Rev. William Chalmers Bird discovered a man naked in the severe winter; and in Pekin we have cold far exceeding anything we get here. He was covered with a cotton quilt, and his two boys, of about ten or twelve years of age, were running about in the keen, bitter north wind, perfectly naked. It was found that opium had brought the father to that state of destitution, for he was an educated man, who could have very easily maintained a good position in China. The man came to me, and I gave him employment, and weaned him from his pipe. He took to it again quietly. I weaned him again. He took to it another time, and at last I was obliged to cast him adrift. After a little time he came to me one day begging. I gave him a meal, and I said, 'You come every day, and I will give you a meal, but I dare not give you money.' He came a second time, and then he pulled aside the only article of clothing that he had on him, and showed me his body covered with sores. I sent him to the hospital of the London Missionary Society, and there he lived a short time; but he died with ulcers inside and outside, a perfect wreck, from smoking opium. I could give you many more instances, but I cannot go on. But remember this, that if we come and bring home this testimony, it is because it has been burnt into our hearts by witnessing, year after year, the destitution and the misery brought upon multitudes in China by this opium.

Why have merchants in China given up the trade—given up what was for their profit? I have known more than one case in which that has been done. I knew a case in which a man who, as far as I know, was not touched by any Christian principle, rejected the profits of the opium because he could not conscientiously take them. Therefore, as

I am speaking now to men who I think sympathize with us in this object, I would simply say, let us go on till, by God's help, we oblige our rulers to look into this matter in the future, and to give up this sad position in which the English Government is the purveyor of a death-dealing poison to China.[1]

The Rev. James Sadler,

Of the London Missionary Society, sixteen years missionary to the Chinese.

My Lord and dear Friends,—I have had considerable opportunity of knowing something of the famine in China; I have been able to see in various places something of the horrors of war and the devastation it has caused; and I have had to do personally with some of the distresses of pestilence. But in my own mind there is a very solemn fear that the distresses in connection with this opium business will be in future, if they are not even at present, greater than the horrors of famine, and the horrors of war, and the horrors of pestilence. I will try to be as brief as possible in giving you a little of my experience of these matters.

THE OPIUM-SMOKER.

First as to the smoker himself. I have seen the man, and I have noticed how he was branded everywhere. The greenish yellow in his eye, the sunken cheek, the emaciated frame, all marked him out, and everybody seemed ashamed of him, as he was ashamed of himself. I have noticed his loss of appetite, and how he had to mince and mess his food in order to get it down in any way. I have noticed his trembling gait, how he seemed under some strong excitement, as though he could hardly walk along; and I have learnt from those who have been intimately acquainted with the matter, how the very functions of nature get out of gear through this horrible habit.

As to the mind, you find that the man is utterly silly and helpless; he seems like a conquered man. Mr. Hill has referred to this matter, and it need not be gone into more fully; but I think that it is a point on which our deepest sympathy ought to be called out. The Chinese have been taken at their weakest point. Heathenism in China just means want of moral power, and this fostering of vice has come in and taken hold of the Chinaman, and he has sunk by degrees to a wretchedness which you cannot find in this country. I wish that all these unhappy

---

[1] I wish to make a few remarks on the statements of Dr. Ayres, as published by the Anti-Opium Society in the pamphlet containing the views of medical men who have been resident in China. Dr. Ayres states that men coming under his charge were at once deprived of the opium they had previously smoked, and that they suffered no ill effects, even though the amount consumed had been two ounces daily; now, I would ask, how did Dr. Ayres discover the amount previously smoked? Of course, as he could not talk Chinese he must have trusted to an interpreter. This system of obtaining information is utterly unreliable. All who know the Chinese are aware that they lie with the utmost appearance of candour and simplicity. Had Dr. Ayres' experience been a tenth part of mine, he must have known that the fact that a man did not suffer, though deprived of even the tenth part of an ounce of opium, which he was said to have smoked, was the most positive proof that he had never smoked opium at all.

wretches, and all those who suffer through them, could be brought and placed in the midst of this Christian country, and then what a feeling of determination would go through all Christian hearts!

HIS FAMILY.

A word or two as to the distress in the family. I have in my mind several families who have suffered from this opium-smoking. In one case a man actually chose his wife because she was clever in making up the opium balls for his pipe. That may set you thinking as to the earthly and sensual tendency of the habit. In one instance, a man was the cause of so much distress to his family, that they had a trouble to find a way of subsistence. And in another case a man had a splendid chance in life, as we are accustomed to put it, but he threw it all away. He threw away education, he threw away his mental power, he threw away his opportunities of a good livelihood, and not only brought himself to misery, but his family suffered with him.

HIS BUSINESS.

Now, a word or two as to the effects upon a man's business. I was thinking yesterday, and I have thought sometimes in moving about the city, how is it that you can carry on such a great amount of trade as you do in this city? Is it not by mutual good faith? This opium-smoking destroys mutual good faith. It takes away a man's character. His word cannot be taken, and you cannot depend upon his being at his work. And so his business is lost. It is a common point, when we are even getting a chair-bearer for our Sedan chairs, to see that the man is not an opium-smoker. If he be, he may let you down in any part of the road, or he may need to go away for a very long time to get his dose.

Then as to the evils in the Church, they are exceedingly great. We have known cases of men who have seemed to get rid of the habit, but it has come upon them again, and has caused continual trouble. Now, as to the difficulties of cure. I said to a man once, 'Why don't you go to the hospital and be cured?' He said, 'How can I? So-and-so went, and in seeking a cure he died. I am not willing to go and die in that way.' Therefore this man objected to go to the hospital. Many of you have seen Dr. Lockhart's opinion in the newspaper. It is very definite from a man who has so much knowledge of China. You remember how he stated that the idea that opium was harmless was entirely wrong. He could not say that opium had become used in China in the same proportion as drink in this country; but then we must not look at the thing in that light. We must observe to what proportions it has already gone, and it is a comparatively new vice in China. What will it be when it shall have existed as long as drunkenness in this country?

You have already heard that the Chinese look at it as an evil. They dread it in their sons and in their servants. They look upon it as amongst the worst forms of wickedness, however fashionable it may be.

WHO IS RESPONSIBLE?

One word as to the question of who is responsible. When we preach in the roadways or in the chapels, or wherever it may be, we are told constantly by the Chinese that we are responsible. You may tell them that they need not purchase opium, and that then it would not be brought. Suppose that some man, unworthy of the name of man, should come and tempt our children into sin, and then should turn round and say, 'Well, they wished to do evil, and it is fashionable to do evil, and men will do evil as long as the world lasts.' Would any of us as parents tolerate a man talking in that way? And so with regard to the Chinese. The vice has been fostered, and now we are to coolly turn round and say, 'Well, they will be wicked, and they must be wicked, and we will help them to be wicked.' I do not know what sort of morality that is. I feel that sometimes there is dust thrown in one's eyes. You hear men talking in a way which makes you fear there is something seriously wrong. Now, I think that we ought always to ask ourselves this question, Is the talk which we hear on behalf of the Chinaman or on behalf of the trade? You must not be surprised if missionaries stand up on behalf of the Chinaman. Would to God that they could be here to stand up for themselves! They 'could a tale unfold.' But the worst of it is, that they are ten thousand miles away, and that is the great difficulty. I find friends saying with regard to the horrors of heathenism, that they cannot understand them, or be impressed by them, because they are so far away. 'Out of sight, out of mind.' But, friends, the evils *do* exist. And now comes the question, How are we to look at this whole question? There are giant evils, and there is giant opposition against the Anti-Opium Society. There is the opposition of gain; there is the opposition of might; there is the opposition of the fact that the evil has been legalized; there is the opposition which arises on the ground of various things connected with heathenism.

But now the one question for us is, Is the power of Christianity or the spirit of Christianity to prove itself a greater power—a more giant energy—than all these things that are against us? Why, it seems to me that what we want now, is not simply that missionaries should represent these things, but that you at home, knowing the facts of the case, should be able to take them up and to create a public opinion concerning the whole traffic. Missionaries want to be away at their work. The point rests with you; that you in England, and all who have any influence or authority in this country, should see what you can do by every possible means to create a public opinion, and to call out the mind of this country so that it shall never rest until the evil is abolished.

The Chairman (Lord Polwarth).

Ladies and Gentlemen,—The meeting is now about to close, and I wish to claim your indulgence for a few minutes. The great object of the meetings which have been held this day, has been to bring before the public of this country the evidence of men who have been in very close contact and intercourse with the Chinese people for a considerable time. I believe that those who are on this platform, and who have spoken here to-night, are men who are thoroughly conversant with the Chinese people; that their calling there has led them to mingle with the people as perhaps no other class of Europeans have had to do; that they have mixed both with the high and with the low, and that they have been able to watch in all its variety the effects of opium in China.

THE TESTIMONY OF MISSIONARIES.

I should just like to refer to one or two points which are before the public at the present time. I often hear it alleged that the testimony of missionaries is to be taken very cautiously in the matter of opium. Why is that? It is stated that missionaries are not trustworthy witnesses in this matter, because opium interferes with the spread of Christianity, which they are there to promote. But what is their one object in China? Is it not the spread of all that tends to morality, to purity, to holiness, to righteousness? And, more than that, may I not claim for Christian missions, wherever they have been, the very highest place as the greatest God-sent influence in civilisation? Wherever Christian missionaries have gone, there have we seen civilisation and industry and art all prospering and flourishing as the result of Christian missions. Therefore I say, that when the missionary contends against the opium trade, it is from motives of the purest philanthropy. He has no other reason. He has no other object in view than, if possible, to bring to an end the traffic which in his eyes, from constant observation, hinders all that is good and noble and true in China.

I believe that we might call together the evidences of missionaries, both Protestant and Catholic, in this respect, and that, if you were to go and ask the teachers of Confucianism themselves whether they would uphold the opium traffic, their answer would be in the negative at once. I believe that we may have evidence from all sides, that the effect of opium on the Chinese population is deleterious and disastrous to the highest degree.

THE OTHER SIDE OF THE QUESTION.

Then I must ask you to look at the other side. There are those who support the opium traffic between India and China. Let us bear and forbear with those who are placed in a somewhat difficult position. There has been handed down to them this particular state of affairs. It is not so easy to shake it off. I believe that it is a very difficult matter so to adjust the affairs of India, and so to adjust taxation, and so to arrange things, as to do without it. I will grant all that; but I think that the opinion of those who are supporting the opium traffic, and of those who are holding office, or who have held office in previous days, has been, that it was impossible to do without the opium trade because they could not do without the money.

But only let the British public realize that the money which is thus obtained is obtained at the cost of the misery and shame and wretchedness of thousands of Chinese, and I think that it will not be long before they will rise up and demand that immediate steps be taken to bring about a thorough change in this respect. I think that we may be encouraged from the very conflict of opinion that is going on in the country on this subject at this moment. It is arousing attention to-day throughout the whole of Great Britain.

THE EVIL NOT REALIZED.

I am sure that there are numbers of people in this country who have no conception of what it is. They do not realize it. I have been contrasting it in my own mind, as I daresay you have been doing, with the awful miseries of drink in this country. Some people say that this opium trade with China does not matter—that it is not worse than the effect of alcohol in this country. But if it is only just as bad, or if it were only half as bad, would it be right for the British nation to have any complicity in forcing it upon another country?

Our position in forcing opium upon China at the first, and in continuing to enforce its entrance into China, is a very serious position for any country to occupy; and I am sure that public opinion is rapidly ripening as to the necessity for withdrawing from a traffic which defiles the conscience of the British nation.

Mr. Donald Matheson.

My Lord, Ladies and Gentlemen,—You have heard the testimony to-night of those medical missionaries who have spoken of the opium traffic. You have heard of the terrible effect of opium upon this great empire of China, and now I think you may state your views as to this subject. I am going to put before you this resolution, which I hope will be unanimously accepted :—

'That this meeting, having heard the testimony of many missionaries long resident in China, and some of whom have travelled far in the interior, is convinced of the disastrous effects of the opium trade, physically, morally, and socially. While acknowledging the financial difficulties surrounding the subject, the meeting is of opinion that it is unworthy of this country to permit the continuance of the opium trade between the Government of India and the Chinese, and that the subject is one claiming the early and earnest consideration of Parliament.'

Mr. T. A. Denny.

My Lord Polwarth, Ladies and Gentlemen,—I have been asked to second the resolution. Ladies and gentlemen of the jury, you have heard the evidence. For my part, I do not want to hear any more evidence. My mind is quite made up. I hope that your minds are quite made up. If you do not believe three hundred and fifty missionaries, and do not believe the Chinese Government, and do not believe the Chinese victims themselves, then whom will you believe?

The fact is, that we are in a very bad state, and the whole thing may be resolved into a word or two, and that is, that we cannot afford to do without this money. That is, the great English nation cannot afford to do what is right. Our Government is just like an eldest son who has succeeded to a very flourishing distillery, and who is awfully troubled in his conscience about making gin; but he says, 'If I do not make the gin, I shall not have the profits;' and so he weighs his conscience in one hand, and the gin and the money in the other; and, as often happens in such cases, the money wins. I believe in my conscience, that the Government are very uncomfortable in this matter, and I do hope and trust that we shall make them more uncomfortable.

As a common-sense man, I do not want an argument to prove to me that morphia, which is a deadly poison, is a good thing. I know that it is not a good thing, and so do you. You know that aconite is not a good thing, do you not? And that these people should three times a day be putting this poison into their systems, and that we should be helping them to do it, surely that is not a very good thing. I do wish that we could afford to do what is right. And I do think it a disastrous thing for this nation to do what is wrong for the sake of money.

I was the other night at a very large party of thieves down Drury Lane (and I do not say this with any disrespect to the present Government), and do you know that the reason that these poor fellows were so dishonest was, that they could not afford to be honest? Well, these poor men, who are the Pariahs of society, and whom we were giving a cup of tea to, had a very good excuse. They had no other resource. But are we to be told that we of this great nation, with India at our back, cannot live without this £7,200,000 which we get from opium? I do not believe one single word of it. I have great pleasure in seconding the resolution.

A GENTLEMAN (speaking from the body of the meeting) said—Mr. Chairman, are the Government in China honest in their desire to do away with opium themselves? At the Society of Arts the other night, the question which the noble Lord put to the speakers, and insisted upon an answer to, was this, 'Is the Government in China really honest in desiring to do away with the opium traffic?' No gentleman here to-night has attempted to answer that question. I am rather surprised at that. I should like some of these China gentlemen who know something of China to tell us whether the Government are really desirous of doing so.

The CHAIRMAN.—I am not aware that there is a representative of the Government of China present here to-night to answer the question, and I am not quite sure that the Government of China has always had a very fair chance to answer.

Mr. MACDONALD.—The Government of China is sincere in their efforts against the evils which afflict the people. Many of the officials smoke opium themselves, but then that does not deprive them of feeling for their country.

The resolution was agreed to.

The Rev. F. W. BALLER.—In answer to that gentleman's question, I would say that the intention of the Chinese Government to suppress the traffic, and its sincerity in desiring its suppression, are shown by the fact that in recent treaties made by them with the United States and with the Government of Russia, opium is prohibited as an article of commerce.

A Gentleman.—It was said that the Government of China had got millions of acres of poppy on their own account. Is that so?

The Rev. F. W. Baller.—No.

Mr. J. E. Mathieson moved a hearty vote of thanks to the chairman for presiding.

Rev. J. McCarthy.—I have very great pleasure in seconding that vote of thanks to his Lordship. I am sure that he could not have been occupied in nobler work than in helping to relieve the Chinese from this terrible curse. With regard to one point which a friend has referred to, I may just say that, having travelled in Western China in 1877, I had an opportunity of seeing vast districts of the country under the cultivation of the poppy to make opium; but wherever I went I found the statement made by the inhabitants, that the cultivation of the poppy is a thing of the *present* generation, and is co-existent with the efforts of the Indian Government to open up a trade route from India into Western China. I would like friends to remember this, in order that they may be able to answer those who say that the Chinese Government are insincere because large tracts of country in China are now under the poppy growth. At this late hour I cannot refer further to this matter.

The motion was carried with acclamation.

Dr. Maxwell and the Rev. J. McCarthy, who were unable, from lack of time, to speak as announced at the meeting, have by request kindly written their statements, which we are glad to be able to give.—Ed.

Testimony of Dr. Maxwell,

Of the English Presbyterian Missionary Society, eight years Medical Missionary in China.

My testimony concerns opium-smoking in the island of Formosa. Formosa, with its three millions of Chinese inhabitants and its few hundred thousands of aborigines, has the repute of being one of the quarters where the vice of opium-smoking is largely practised. And the charge is true; true, that is to say, so far as it concerns the Chinese, for amongst the civilised aborigines the practice of opium-smoking is by no means common, and amongst the savages it is unknown. In Formosa, as on the opposite mainland, it should be remembered, however, that even among the Chinese it is in the cities and towns and large villages that the power and ravages of the vice are chiefly seen. The agricultural population in the smaller villages and hamlets are comparatively free from the evil, a state of things which harmonizes at once the clear and reiterated statements of a multitude of witnesses, as to the terrible extent of the vice, and the misery produced by it; and the statistics of Mr. Hart, the Inspector-

General of Customs, who, arguing from the whole 400 millions of China, minimizes the mischief by calculations which seek to prove that there cannot, after all, be more than a few millions of opium-smokers in the empire.

STEADY GROWTH OF OPIUM-SMOKING.

A far more important matter is to be aware of the steady growth of the vice, and this we can do with small risk of error, by looking at the Customs returns, which show the quantity of the drug which enters China from year to year. At the beginning of the century the annual quantity sent forward from India amounted to about 5000 chests; it is now close upon 90,000 chests, or about 6000 tons of opium. There is no possible mistake about this calculation; and if we add that, since the legalization of the import by the treaty of 1860, the native growth of opium has advanced from small beginnings to a trade which now vies in extent with the East Indian trade, it will be seen that the actual increase of opium consumption has been sufficient to warrant the gravest apprehension for the future of China.

OPIUM-SMOKING A DEADLY VICE.

I have called the practice of opium-smoking a vice. I do not hesitate to say that it is a deadly vice, ruinous alike to the moral and physical wellbeing of the man who is enslaved by it. In using such language, I am only speaking in harmony with the universal sentiment of the Chinese themselves in South-Eastern China, the portion of the empire in which I have lived.

As a habit, opium-smoking stands in a category by itself. It is never classed with either tobacco-smoking or spirit-drinking. Tobacco-smoking is universal in China. Men and women alike indulge in it, but nobody dreams of characterizing the practice as vicious. Spirit-drinking is common, but it is not to excess. You very rarely, if ever, meet a drunken Chinaman, and nobody in China thinks of characterizing the use of spirit as a vicious and ruinous habit. It is very different with opium-smoking. The moral sense of the Chinaman, the ordinary average Chinaman, recognises in it a deadly evil. Even the men who are in the clutches of the habit do not hesitate, in their sober moments, to speak of it as a curse. Why is this? If opium-smoking, as Sir George Birdwood alleges, is not a whit more hurtful than smoking willow leaves, or anything else that no one ever dreams of as hurtful, why should the Chinaman speak of it as a curse? Why should fathers and mothers regard their sons as lost to them when they have yielded to the seductions of opium? Why should wives regard with horror the formation of the habit by their husbands? Could not Sir George reassure them, by scientific proof, that the morphia in the prepared opium is non-volatilizable, and that opium-smoking is as innocuous as 'twiddling one's thumbs'? Tens of thousands, alas! of ruined characters, and tens of thousands of ruined homes, are the sad answer to such intolerable nonsense from a scientific defender of the traffic. What matters it to the Chinese whether morphia is volatilizable or not, if the ruin is still the same? I have myself pleaded with men, fine lovable fellows, in good positions, to whom I was indebted for personal kindnesses, men on whom the mark of the opium tyranny was becoming all too visible; I have pleaded with them to give up the habit, which they themselves acknowledged was exercising a growingly evil influence upon them. Why should I have been such a fool? Is not the morphia in the prepared opium non-volatilizable?

My first location in Formosa was in a seaport village with from 2000 to 3000 inhabitants. In that little place, I am sorry to say, there were more opium shops than rice or provision shops; and it was painful to see, especially among the lowest class of labourers, the number of thin sallow faces, which had their origin in opium-smoking. During the *first four months* of dispensary work in Ta-kao, I found that, out of a total of 649 patients, including women and children, there were 247 opium-smokers. Of these 247, 109 presented themselves expressly for assistance to overcome and get rid of the habit. I do not, of course, say that all of these 109 were animated by the purest of motives in their request. Some were under the pressure of poverty, and, having a family dependent upon them, were anxious to do without an article which was a heavy drain on the purse. Some came, doubtless, at the instigation of friends, who saw the increasing danger ahead; some were discontented with the amount of time consumed in the practice; and a fair number were stirred by a hearty desire to be rid of a habit which they felt to be entirely evil. A year or two later I settled in Tai-wan Fu, the capital of the island, a city of between 100,000 and 200,000 inhabitants, and I noted that, in the *first five months*, 250 persons appealed to me, seeking a cure for opium-smoking. This record of only a few months shows how fearfully prevalent the practice was in that community. Indeed, the Chinese themselves put the opium-smokers down as forming a half, or at least a third, of the adult male population in the city. And the eagerness to secure help to overcome it, showed, to some extent at least, how far the smokers themselves were from regarding the habit as innocuous.

Amongst working-men—and my dealings were for the most part with such—the most visible evidence of opium-smoking is emaciation. With wages at a shilling a day, or a little less, the day-labourer who surrenders himself to the opium pipe does not fail, ere long, to spend the major portion of his earnings on the pipe. He will rather stint the food than the drug; and the impaired nutrition consequent on the use of the pipe, coupled with the limited food, speedily shows itself in loss of flesh. If a slight stress comes, either from sickness or diminished earnings, the result in the way of loss of flesh becomes still more apparent, and great numbers of these poor men succumb at an early period to attacks of disease, fever, dysentery, etc., which non-smokers easily overcome.

OPIUM-SMOKING NOT PREVENTIVE OF DISEASE.

I believe that it is an utter delusion to regard opium-smoking in China as a preventive of disease. If careful statistics could be compiled, I should be intensely surprised if they did not reveal that opium-smokers are far more susceptible of disease, and far more liable to succumb to it, than those who do not smoke opium. I have treated many opium-smokers for malarial fever, the one disease which the defenders of the trade love to adduce as being remarkably ameliorated or prevented by its use. I remember that almost the only occasion on which I suffered an opium pipe to be used within my hospital premises, was to mitigate the misery of a man who made a last effort and crawled to the hospital for assistance. He was so far gone with malarial fever that nothing could be done for him but to put him on a bed for the hour or two which he had yet to live. Poor fellow! Even then the opium craving came upon him with intense power, and he entreated me to let him have a pipe. I could not refuse him, and sent in to the landlord of my hospital premises, who himself kept an opium shop, explaining the circumstances, and begging the loan of an opium pipe. The answer was, that the opium might be had for purchase, but no pipe could be loaned off the premises. Happily there was another opium shop close by, the landlord of which had been a patient of mine on several occasions, and who gave me what I wanted, so that the opium-hunger of the dying man was satisfied.

OPIUM-SMOKING MORE DANGEROUS THAN SPIRIT-DRINKING.

The grievous danger of the vice of opium-smoking lies in the quiet and insidious way in which it lays hold of those who dally with it. Not only is there an entire absence of the brutality and violence which characterize even a first over-indulgence in alcohol, but there is also an initiatory period, in which there is either no craving, or the craving is so slight that it can be resisted without much effort. Indeed, there are certainly not a few in China, merchants and others, who may now and again smoke the opium pipe, but who are wise enough to beware of the daily habit. When the daily habit is entered upon, a few weeks are sufficient to make the effort to throw off the chain so severe a tax, alike on the physical and moral strength of a man, that without help he rarely comes off the victor. It is this insidious and quiet and comparatively speedy way in which it takes firm hold of its victim that renders opium-smoking so much more dangerous a vice in many respects than spirit-drinking. It is far quicker in its capture of the man, and more difficult to be shaken off, even when the will is roused to attempt it. Happily, with the help of a physician, and with the patient secluded from the possibility of temptation, there are not a few cases where a cure has been effected.

THE CHINESE WISH TO PUT DOWN OPIUM-SMOKING.

Are the Chinese honest, it is asked, in their expressions of desire to restrain and put down this immense evil in the empire? I believe they are. We who have brought them into their present position, and who keep them there, have least of all a right to question their truth in this matter. In the eyes of Chinese people and rulers alike, opium-smoking is a vice, and is condemned as such. At present, all clear and definite action to shake themselves free from it is forbidden by the treaty with England. They cannot prevent opium coming in at every one of their open ports; and ever since the treaty of 1860, which legalized such import, the Government of China has had no moral standing from which to combat the native growth. If it is right to allow the foreigners to bring it and sell it everywhere on the coast, what wrong can there be in growing it in China itself? Even whilst the national sentiment distinctly condemns the vice of opium-smoking, national pride and national cupidity say, 'We need not let the foreigner have it all his own way.' They palliate the more readily, at least, the action of those who assert this right and act upon it, even though it is to the detriment of high national interests.

POWER OF THE CHINESE TO PUT DOWN OPIUM-SMOKING.

Can the Chinese, it is further asked, put down the vice if they were free to try? Again, why should we doubt it? If an active viceroy can in his province, as recently in Shan-si, utterly put down the growth of the poppy even for a year or two, why not for a longer period, and why not throughout the empire? If Li Hung-chang at Tientsin, or Tan Tse-tso at Soo-chow, can shut up every opium den in these great cities, and limit opium-smoking to private houses, confiscating right and left the property of any man who dares to defy their rules; and if they can carry this on for years, and what is more, have the heart of the population with them in these attempts to restrain and diminish this sore evil,—what right have we to assume that, with more power in their hands, such men and leaders could not inaugurate an opium reform in China worthy of the truest patriotism? Great cities are a crucial test in such a question, and these men have shown what can be done.

Why, again, has China, in her recently concluded treaties with the United States, Brazil, and Russia, made a point of debarring the possibility of an opium trade on the part of these countries, if she is not anxious to restrain and put down the traffic; and if her Government did not feel that only the treaty obligations with England limited her power to do for her people what she would desire to do in this matter?

It is surely an unholy revenue that blinds men's eyes to some of the plainest dictates of fairness and honour in our dealings as a nation with China in this matter. Whatever men may say, such a revenue is a continuous curse.

TESTIMONY OF REV. J. McCARTHY,

Of the China Inland Mission, twelve years missionary in China.

My testimony concerning opium is based upon an experience of twelve years in China. During these years I lived among the people, and had familiar intercourse with them day by day, and thus had opportunity to observe the effects of opium-smoking. I cannot speak with the scientific knowledge of the medical missionary, nor is it needful that I should. A long course of medical training is not necessary to enable any one to know that in this country drunkenness is a great source of misery, wretchedness, and crime. In like manner, one who has lived in China is able to see that opium-smoking is a source of untold sorrow and ruin. If in England a man professed, on scientific or any other principles, to prove that drunkenness, so far from being a curse, was really a harmless indulgence, a help and comfort, the one recreation of the average Englishman, he would be laughed at as a harmless person, for whom his friends should be made responsible, and would be likely to provoke feelings of regret, or even of anger, if his statements proved to be a hindrance to the work of those who were seeking to mitigate the evils arising from our drink traffic. Those who have lived among the Chinese—not merely been *to* China, or lived *in* China, but whose lives have been spent among the people—find it very difficult to suppress their feelings of wonder and indignation when they find the plainest facts of their every-day experience as foolishly questioned or denied.

From the very nature of things, men of ordinary mental capacity would be prepared to believe that the habitual use of a poisonous drug *could* only be injurious, and actual experience of the facts in the case of opium, places this beyond question.

That opium merchants or Government officials should be prepared to advance statements which seem to favour the circumstances in which they find themselves (circumstances which are so profitable), with our knowledge of human nature, does not seem a very wonderful thing. But neither opium merchants nor Government officials have facilities for knowing, from personal observation, the evils of opium-smoking, such as are possessed by the youngest or most inexperienced missionary. Merchants and traders *will not*, and Government officials, from their very position, *cannot* mix freely with the people, and consequently are not in a position directly to get the facts of the case.

The fact that a man has sold twenty thousand chests of opium through a middle-man, to whom he speaks in a jargon called 'pidgin' (business) English, does not place him in a position to deny the evils which missionaries, in their every-day intercourse with the people, see to be flowing from each one of these twenty thousand chests. These, and like considerations, must be borne in mind when balancing evidence on this question.

THE UNIVERSAL TESTIMONY OF THE CHINESE.

The universal testimony of the heathen Chinese is, that mentally, morally, and physically, opium-smoking is most pernicious in its effects. Parents consider it the greatest calamity that can befall them or their families, that any of their children should begin the habit of opium-smoking. I knew a well-authenticated case, where a father, having warned and expostulated with, and repeatedly helped an opium-smoking son without effect, at length put him in a sack and drowned him in the canal which flowed through the village, *with the approval of the whole community*, and solely because the son was considered a hopeless opium-smoker.

The people assert freely and believe firmly, that the number of children born to opium-smokers is less than to other men, and that it thus tends to reduce the population.

They give you circumstantial accounts of prospects blighted, of families ruined, and lives shortened through the indulgence by one or more members of a family in this habit.

To the use of the 'foreign medicine' (opium) are traced evils only to be at all approached by the sad and dreary catalogue which we get on every hand in connection with the drinking customs of our own land.

Papers and pamphlets written by the Chinese themselves are distributed, in which the physical and intellectual and moral evils connected with opium-smoking are vividly described, and the young especially warned against the habit.

It is always spoken of as a *vice*, being classed with gambling, stealing, adultery, murder, etc.

The opium-smoker himself generally seeks to hide the fact as long as it is possible. He feels ashamed to own that he is learning to indulge in a habit which on all hands is acknowledged to do such harm. It is also contrary to his feelings of respect for his forefathers that he should thus injure the body which they have given him.

When the habit becomes fixed, the family of the opium-smoker may accept the evil as one that must be endured, and then the smoking is more above board, but it is almost always spoken of with regret, and as a necessity on account of ill-health, or, it may be, from inability to give up a bad practice begun in youth. During my twelve years' experience, spent in different parts of China, I have only met with *one* Chinaman who attempted to defend the practice of opium-smoking, and on *that account* he was considered even by his friends as pre-eminently a worthless fellow.

The Chinese Christians, many of whom have, through God's blessing on the use of medicines, been rescued from the habit, are also unanimous in their opinion as to the degrading and demoralizing effects of opium-smoking, and refuse to receive into church-fellowship any indulging in the drug. To begin to smoke opium would expose a man, already a church-member, to expulsion; the Christians feel that that which even the heathen look upon as a vice cannot be tolerated within the Church. Though it may often be difficult to bring home the fact to the opium-smoker, who seeks to hide that he indulges in the practice, yet it is never difficult to *know* that he smokes opium. His face, manner, and general appearance betray his condition to the natives, or to any who have had experience, and who give attention to the subject. It is not at all necessary to be a medical man in order to know an opium-smoker.

OPIUM-SMOKING AND INTOXICATING DRINK.

There need be no hesitation in saying that opium-smoking is much worse than ordinary drinking at home. Opium-smoking should not be classed with drinking merely, but with *intoxication*. *Many* men, who drink a little continually, are yet never intoxicated; but the percentage of opium-smokers who are not *slaves* to the pipe is so small that it may be said not to exist. Even in the case of those who have not become the victims of the opium craving, the limited use even of the drug leaves the system in such a condition, that it is a well-known fact that such opium-smokers will die of a disease that an ordinary person will get through easily. And it must be remembered that what, for want of a better title, is called *moderate* opium-smoking in the vast majority of cases must become immoderate, *does* in fact become so, and that from the very nature of the effect of the drug upon the system, which leads the victim to crave for more and more in order to produce the desired effect.

We are not confined, however, either to the testimony of missionaries to China, or the Chinese themselves, as to the evils of opium-smoking. The baneful effects of opium-smoking upon the native population in Burmah has been so injurious, and so notorious, that Government action has been taken to close some of the opium dens, and thus in some measure stay the evil. If it has proved such a curse in the low, marshy, aguish districts of Lower Burmah, how can it be spoken of as a benefit in the high table-lands or extensive plains which form the greater part of China?

Can missionaries, then, reasonably be charged as fanatics if they express an opinion that England should not be in any way a party to the growth and production of a drug which, used as it is in China, causes such dire results?

Should missionaries be charged with exaggeration when they say, that it is deplorable that a professedly Christian nation should in the past have insisted upon the introduction of opium into China?

And are missionaries unreasonable when they ask, 'Can anything really be said in defence of a policy which refuses to allow China to be free in the matter of admitting or not admitting this drug into her territory?'

Opium, as an intoxicant, *is* a pernicious drug. It *is* causing untold misery in China. It would be very difficult to exaggerate the evils which result from its use. But I am free to say, that if we had used the means we have used for the introduction of opium for the introduction of chairs and tables into China, our action would be equally indefensible. If we had deliberately set ourselves—as we have never done—to introduce Bibles into China in the same way that, as a nation, we have set ourselves to introduce opium, I say unhesitatingly our action would have been equally indefensible. We have no right, at the point of the bayonet, to *compel* others to receive even that which we believe would be a benefit to them. Such conduct might be worthy the followers of the False Prophet, but would be quite incompatible with allegiance to Jesus of Nazareth. How *much more* heinous must such a course be when it is a traffic in an article which *can* only bring ruin and misery!

SINCERITY OF THE CHINESE.

But some say, 'The Chinese are not sincere in their desire to put down the opium traffic.' We ask any who really think so to read the history of the question, and then to suggest any way in which a nation could more clearly show its anxiety to rid itself of an intolerable burden than the way the Chinese have adopted, bearing in mind the fact that China was a weak power, and that England was a strong power, and that while at war with us China had to deal with internal rebellions, which crippled her resources.

Others say, 'They grow opium themselves; all over Western China large tracts of land are under poppy cultivation;' and they ask, 'How can the Chinese be sincere in their desire to get rid of opium when they grow it themselves?' Our friends who so strenuously urge this objection always fail to state the fact, however, that the extensive growth of opium in China is a thing of the present generation.

In 1877 I travelled across the country into Burmah. On every hand in Si-chuan, and Kwei-chau, and Yun-nan, I found the poppy largely cultivated, but everywhere found, upon conversation with the people, that its cultivation had been begun within the memory of middle-aged men. Before that time patches here and there had doubtless been grown, but not in such quantity, or on such a scale, as to be of any serious moment.

The period of the persistent effort of England—our *successful* effort to introduce the drug on the Eastern seaboard, and our continued though *unsuccessful* efforts to open up a trade route from India into China on the West—will really cover the period of time during which opium has been so largely grown in China. Could we blame the Chinese Government if, failing to induce us to remove our pressure, and stop or reduce our import of opium into their country, they should, in very despair, seek to put us out of the market by allowing their own people to produce the drug? Indeed, while *compelled* to receive our opium, we can scarcely imagine that the Chinese authorities could use their power to carry out the restrictions already in force against the growth of the poppy; so that for the native growth of opium, as well as for that imported, we must be held largely responsible. The best men, the most powerful men in China, *are* opposed to the growth of opium, and are determined to put it down. The task would be difficult, but few who have had any experience of the power of the central government to carry out its wishes all over the empire, can doubt that the men who are now at the head of affairs in China, *could* put down the poppy cultivation, if the outside pressure were removed. And there is every reason to believe that they would honestly make the attempt. Whether they succeeded or not, they ought to be left free to put in force their so oft-repeated professions. It is *wicked* to charge them with insincerity while we refuse to allow them to prove their sincerity.

INDIA AND THE OPIUM REVENUE.

But the question is also gravely asked, 'What are we to do in India without this opium revenue?' 'It may be a crime to force the Chinese to have our opium, we may lament the misery caused by the use of that opium in China; but however trying to our feelings all this may be, we really *do* need the money in India; in fact, we cannot do without it.' The British nation—the great British nation—can only maintain its hold over the millions of India by doing what it can to poison the millions of China! Alas! how are the mighty fallen! 'Get money, honestly if you can, but *get* it, for you need it.' This may be devil's doctrine, but it is not doctrine worthy of a great and Christian nation like England. And yet something like this in effect is often urged, and that by men who ought to know better. The God of nations, who loves the Chinese people as well as the people of these isles, can easily blow upon, and scatter, all ill-gotten gains; and it is easy for us, by wars, and famine, and pestilence, to lose far more than we appear to gain by our opium revenue.

Looking at the matter from our opponents' point of view, we may ask them, 'What will they do for revenue when China refuses to have any more of our opium? Will England again go to war to force this poison upon China?' We may with confidence say—NEVER. I have faith in the power of truth, and the *facts* of this opium business need only to be *known* in order to prevent such a possibility, and to secure a settlement of the question for ever. They are the truest friends of the Indian Government who urge upon them the propriety of finding some other source of revenue besides that from opium; for it is all but certain that, if our country does not relieve China from the pressure of our opium traffic, China will take the matter into its own hands, and settle the question in a way that will not be so agreeable to us, before long.

If we are wise, and seek to rid ourselves of this traffic, as far as we can, thus trying to repair the evil we have done (which, alas! is really impossible), it may give us a legacy of kindly feeling and goodwill in the minds of the Chinese, which will be for our own benefit for generations yet to come, while if the matter is taken in hand and settled by the Chinese Government, the odium and disgrace will be ours to the end of time.

Testimony of Rev. Griffith John,

Of the London Missionary Society, twenty-six years missionary in China.

England has been the means of opening the Chinese empire to the merchants of the world, and it is our duty as a Christian nation to take a deep interest in its highest prosperity. Moreover, our connection with China has not been a source of unmixed blessing to the people.

UNSPEAKABLE EVILS OF THE OPIUM TRADE.

Think of the opium trade, and of the unspeakable evils which it has brought upon that land! The Chinese call us devils, and when I think of this unprincipled and destructive trade, I cease to wonder at it. Previous to the year 1767, the opium trade was almost entirely in the hands of the Portuguese; but the quantity annually imported did not exceed 200 chests. In 1773, we find the East India Company in the field as importers of the drug; and under its auspices and fostering care the trade grew rapidly, so as to reach in 1854 as much as 78,354 chests. I cannot now go over the sad history of the shameful trade, nor describe the selfish conduct of the British Government in respect to it. It is well known that the attempt made by the Emperor Tau-kwang to put an end to the traffic was the immediate cause of our first war with China. That war cost the Chinese 21,000,000 dols. and the island of Hong-kong, to say nothing of the great losses and evils it brought with it to the empire. For the destroyed opium we compelled the Chinese to pay 6,000,000 dols. When all was over, our plenipotentiary, Sir H. Pottinger, did what he could to persuade the Chinese to legalize the traffic. But what was the emperor's reply? 'It is true,' said he, 'I cannot prevent the introduction of the flowing poison; gain-seeking and corrupt men will, for profit and sensuality, defeat my wishes; but nothing will induce me to derive a revenue from the vice and misery of my people.' Noble words! They are worthy of being written in letters of gold. To my mind, the heathen monarch stood on a much higher moral platform than the Christian plenipotentiary. The next thing Great Britain did, through Lord Elgin, was to persuade the Chinese Government to legalize the traffic, and thus cause opium-smoking to become a safe, respectable, and general practice over the length and breadth of the land.

The Chinese pay us for this destructive poison from £14,000,000 to £16,000,000 per annum; whilst the value of the British produce exported from the United Kingdom to China is only from £8,000,000 to £10,000,000. Such is the position of Great Britain, the representative of Christianity in the East, in China as a great commercial country. But opium is not only robbing the Chinese of millions of money year by year, but is actually destroying them as a people. It undermines the constitution, ruins the health, and shortens the life of the smoker; destroys every domestic happiness and prosperity; and is gradually affecting the physical, mental, and moral deterioration of the nation as a nation. The Chinese tell us that a large proportion of the regular opium-smokers are childless, and that the children of the others are few, feeble, and sickly. They also affirm that the family of the opium-smoker will be extinct in the third generation.

When a man smokes, his son generally smokes also, and begins at an earlier age than his father did; so that if the son be not childless, as is often the case, his children are born with feeble constitutions, and die prematurely. Our merchants and Government may speak of the opium trade as a 'political necessity,' and as being 'regulated by the ordinary laws of supply and demand.' That is one way of looking at it, and a very soothing way, I suppose, to those who are interested in it. But the Chinese themselves say that 'England trades in opium because she desires to work China's ruin.' 'It is not only,' writes one of the natives, 'that year by year they abstract so many millions of our money, but the direful appearances seem to indicate a wish on their part to utterly root out and extirpate us as a nation.' Some tell us that the use of opium is not a curse, but a comfort and a benefit to the hardworking Chinese; and one has been assuring the public recently that opium-smoking is as innocuous as the 'twiddling of one's thumbs.' How to deal with statements of this kind, it is difficult to see. To one who has lived in the country for twenty-six years, they appear utterly unaccountable. I would not in any case put them down to wilful misrepresentation; and yet it is difficult to ascribe them in some cases to ignorance.

OPIUM-SMOKING AN UNMITIGATED CURSE.

All that I wish to affirm is, that they are wholly false, and that opium-smoking in China, so far from being an innocent enjoyment, is an unmitigated curse to both the nation and the individual. The missionary is made to feel constantly that this pernicious trade, with its disgraceful history, speaks more eloquently and convincingly to the Chinese mind against Christianity than he does or can do for it. The trade has created a strong prejudice against the missionary and the gospel. The Chinese cannot understand how the same people can bring to them a gospel of salvation in one hand, and a destructive poison in the other. They do not see how it is possible for us to feel such a tremendous interest in their souls, whilst we are destroying their bodies by the million; and they have their doubts as to whether a people who could carry on such a traffic have a right to talk to them about religion, and exhort them to virtue. Though we as missionaries are free from the abomination, the Chinese cannot draw the line of demarcation. And then they will ask: 'Is this trade a legitimate fruit of Christianity?' But, granting that Christianity is not responsible for it, and that it is carried on in spite of Christ's golden rule,—to do unto others as we would have others do unto us,—what is the use of Christianity if this trade is a specimen of its influence on the hearts and lives of men? It is useless to say that the Chinese are growing opium themselves, and that they will continue to do so, whether we import it or not. We have nothing to do with the possible or probable action of the Chinese in the matter. It is for us to wash our hands clean of the iniquity, and allow them to deal with it as they please. The trade is immoral, and a foul blot on England's escutcheon. It is not for us to perpetrate murder in order to prevent the Chinese from committing suicide. It is, however, by no means certain that the Chinese would not make an honest effort to stop the native growth, if we would only give them a fair chance to do so, by stopping the importation. I believe they would make the attempt, though I am not prepared to promise that the result would be satisfactory. I cannot close my eyes to the fact that opium-smoking in China has become so common, and that the habit has such a hold on its victim, that in my most calm and solemn moments, I can see no hope except in God. There are millions in China to whom the drug is dearer than life itself. Even if the foreign trade in the drug were given up, it is more than probable that opium-smoking, and consequently opium-growing, would go on in the provinces. Yun-nan, Kwei-chau, and Si-chuan are red with the poppy every year; whilst in several of the other provinces it is extensively cultivated.

The evil is now one of enormous magnitude; and I am inclined to think that no legislative measures on the part of the Chinese Government, however honestly adopted, will put an end to it. Be that as it may, our path as a Christian nation is plain enough. We have inflicted a terrible wrong on the people of China, and it is our solemn duty to try and undo it, by abandoning the trade at once and for ever ourselves, and by giving them every sympathy and aid in our power in their attempt to banish the curse from within their own borders. Would to God it were possible to bring the British Government to see the wicked character of the traffic, and to induce them to 'sacrifice their opium revenue on the altar of our national Christianity and China's wellbeing!'—*From 'China: her Claims and Call.'*

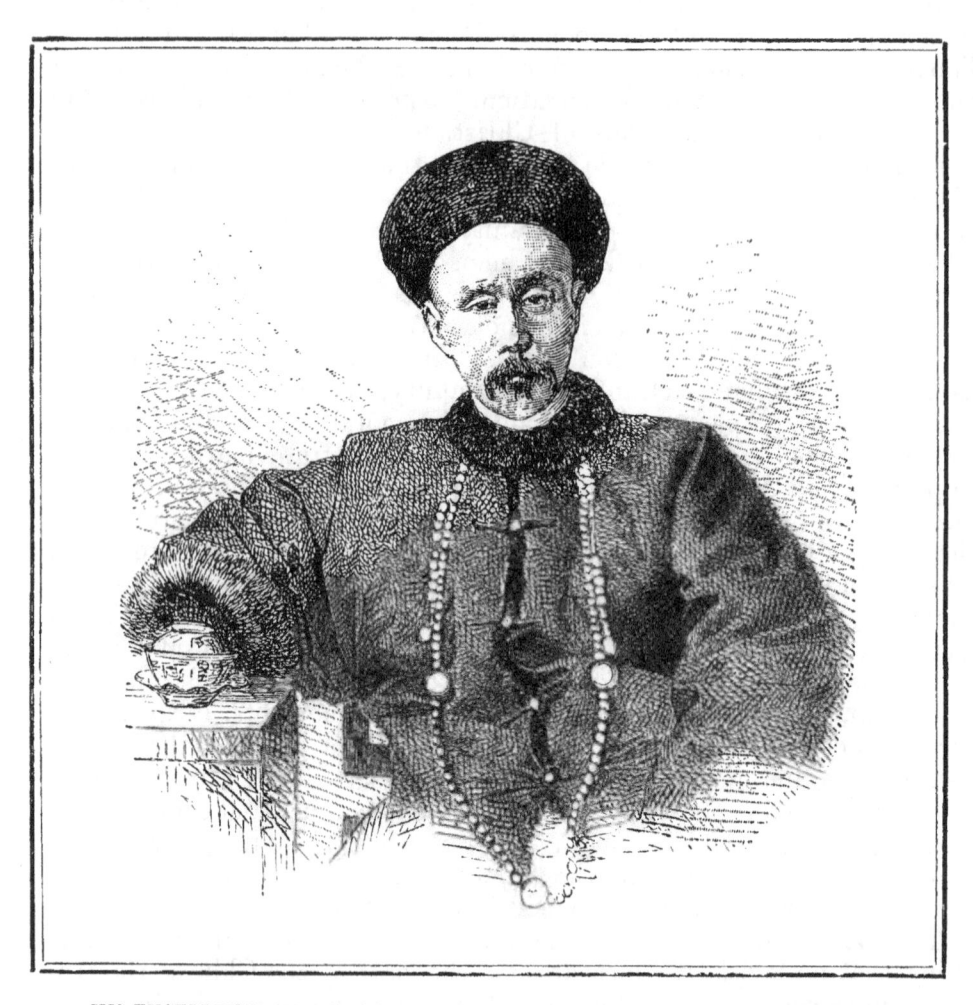

HIS EXCELLENCY THE GRAND SECRETARY AND VICEROY, LI HUNG-CHANG.

APPENDIX.

EXCUSES FOR THE OPIUM TRADE.

Excuse 1.—THAT OPIUM-SMOKING IS NOT VERY INJURIOUS.

That opium is very injurious is abundantly proved :—(1) By what the Chinese have done and said concerning it. (2) By the testimony of Sir Rutherford Alcock, and other officials. (3) By the unanimous testimony of all missionaries. And (4) by the almost universal testimony of medical men.

TESTIMONY OF THE CHINESE.

SIR RUTHERFORD ALCOCK, K.C.B.,

Her Majesty's Representative in China, in his evidence before the House of Commons Committee on East India Finance in 1871, said :—

'5694. *A.* I should be very glad if you would allow me to read some passages from my despatch [to Lord Clarendon] on that subject, because it states in the shortest possible way with what view the Chinese Government were then pressing, in fact, for the total prohibition of opium, as being *too injurious to them to be tolerated or endured.*'

In this despatch, Sir Rutherford gives an account of his conversation with some of the leading members of the Foreign Office at Pekin. The following brief extract shows the Chinese estimate of the evil of opium-smoking :—

'PEKIN, *May* 24*th*, 1869.

'From missionary troubles and dangers, the conversation diverged to the hostile animus which was so constantly manifested by the literati, and all the official class, against foreigners generally, irrespective of religious questions. . . .

'In the end Wen-seang shifted his ground; and, after first maintaining the innocence of the party accused, he admitted that there might be some of the literati who were imbued with a hostile feeling; but, he asked, how could it be otherwise? and proceeded to put in a plea of justification, saying they had often seen foreigners making war on the country; and then, again, *how irreparable and continuous was the injury which they inflicted upon the whole empire by the foreign importation of opium.*

'He then added, if England would consent to interdict this,—cease either to grow it in India, or to allow their ships to bring it to China,—there might be some hope of more friendly feelings. No doubt there was a very strong feeling entertained by all the literati and gentry as to *the frightful evils attending the smoking of opium, its thoroughly demoralizing effects, and the utter ruin brought upon all who once gave way to the vice.* He believed the extension of this pernicious habit was mainly due to the alacrity with which foreigners supplied the poison for their own profit, perfectly *regardless of the irreparable injury inflicted*, and naturally they felt hostile to all concerned in such a traffic.' . . .

'Subsequent to this conference, I received, in the month of June, from the Foreign Board of Peking, an official note urging upon Her Majesty's Government the policy of prohibiting the importation of foreign opium, as being prejudicial to the general interests of commerce. As the memorial is but a short one, I think it would be satisfactory to the Committee if I read it, instead of giving a mere abstract.'

This memorial from the Government of China is a most important document. It shows how deeply the leading officials of the Empire felt the evils consequent upon the opium trade, and how earnestly they entreated the British authorities to do away with it.

Mr. Henry Richard, M.P., truly described it when he said it was 'a powerful and pathetic appeal from the Chinese to the conscience and kindly feeling of the British nation.' And Sir R. Alcock, after reading it to the House of Commons Committee, said, 'I think that the Committee will see that this is a very significant document.'

Memorial from the Government of China.

'From Tsung-li Yamen to Sir R. Alcock, July 1869.—The writers have on several occasions, when conversing with His Excellency the British Minister, referred to the opium trade as being prejudicial to the general interests of commerce. The object of the treaties between our respective countries was to secure perpetual peace; but if effective steps cannot be taken to remove an accumulating sense of injury from the minds of men, it is to be feared that no policy can obviate sources of future trouble.

'Day and night the writers are considering the question with a view to its solution, and the more they reflect upon it, the greater does their anxiety become, and hereon they cannot avoid addressing His Excellency very earnestly on the subject.

'That opium is like *a deadly poison*, that *it is most injurious to mankind*, and a most serious provocative of ill-feeling, is, the writers think, perfectly well known to His Excellency, and it is therefore needless for them to enlarge further on these points. The prince' (the Prince of Kung is the president of the Board) 'and his colleagues are quite aware that the opium trade has long been condemned by England as a nation, and that the right-minded merchant scorns to have to do with it.

PRINCE KUNG.   WEN-SEANG.

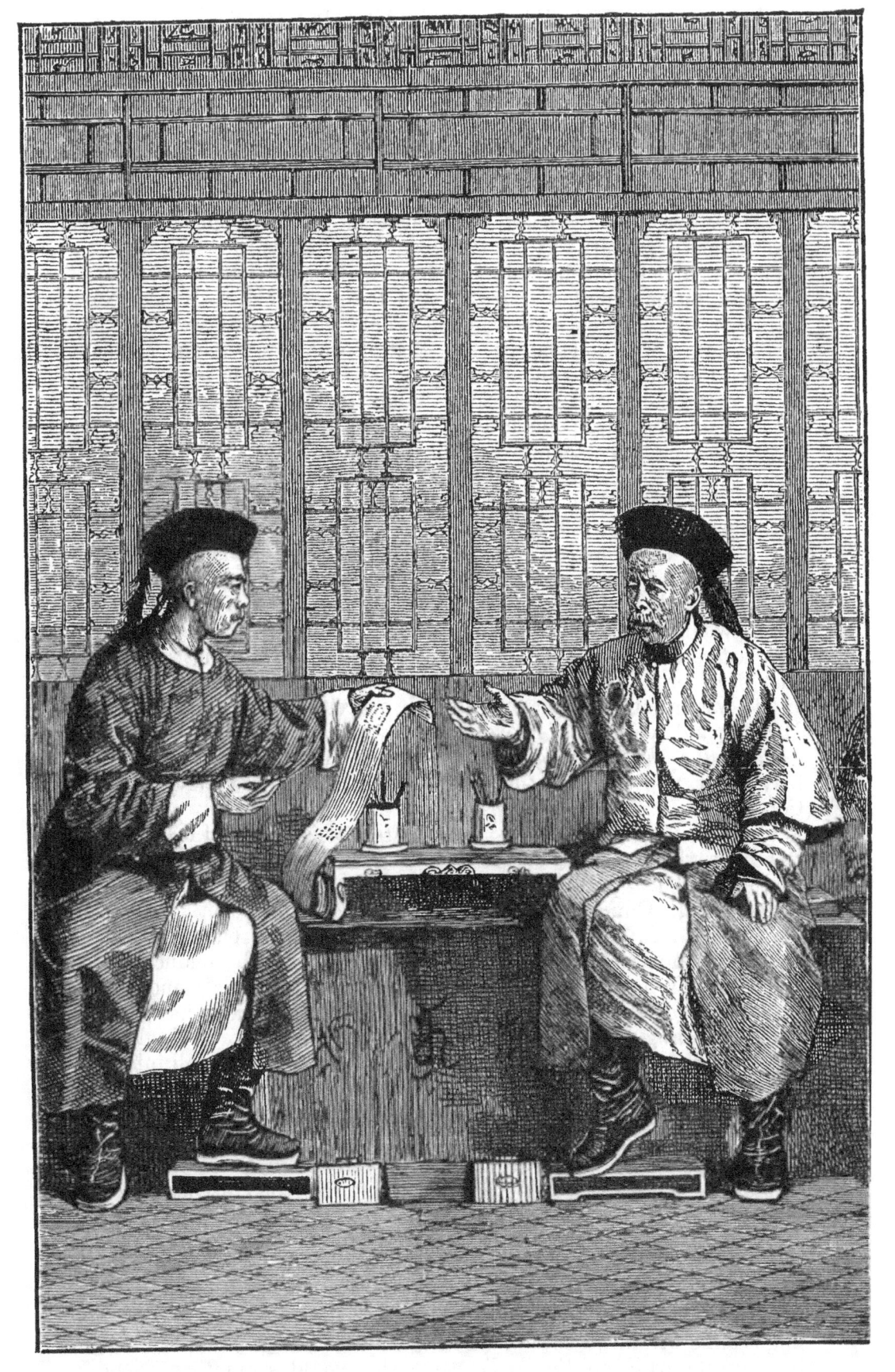

'But the officials and people of this empire, who cannot be so completely informed on the subject, all say that England trades in opium because she desires to work China's ruin, for (say they) if the friendly feelings of England are genuine, since it is open to her to produce and trade in everything else, would she still insist on spreading *the poison of this hurtful thing through the empire?*

'There are those who say, stop the trade by enforcing a vigorous prohibition against the use of the drug. China has the right to do so, doubtless, and might be able to effect it; but a strict enforcement of the prohibition would necessitate the taking of many lives. Now, although the criminals' punishment would be of their own seeking, bystanders would not fail to say that it was the foreign merchant seduced them to their ruin by bringing the drug, and it would be hard to prevent general and deep-seated indignation; such a course, indeed, would tend to arouse popular anger against the foreigner.

'There are others, again, who suggest the removal of the prohibitions against the growth of the poppy. They argue that, as there is no means of stopping the foreign (opium) trade, there can be no harm, as a temporary measure, in withdrawing the prohibition on its growth. We should thus not only deprive the foreign merchant of a main source of his profits, but should increase our revenue to boot. The sovereign rights of China are, indeed, competent to this. Such a course would be practicable; and, indeed, the writers cannot say that, as a last resource, it will not come to this; but they are most unwilling that such prohibition should be removed, holding, as they do, that a right system of government should appreciate the beneficence of Heaven, and (seek to) remove any grievance which afflicts its people, *while, to allow them to go on to destruction*, although an increase of revenue may result, will provoke the judgment of Heaven and the condemnation of men.

'Neither of the above plans, indeed, are satisfactory. If it be desired to remove the very root, and to stop the evil at its source, nothing will be effective but a prohibition, to be enforced alike by both parties.

'Again, the Chinese merchant supplies your country with his goodly tea and silk, conferring thereby a benefit upon her; but the English merchant empoisons China with *pestilent opium*. Such conduct is unrighteous. Who can justify it? What wonder if officials and people say that *England is wilfully working out China's ruin*, and has no real friendly feeling for her? The wealth and generosity of England is spoken of by all; she is anxious to prevent and anticipate all injury to her commercial interest. How is it, then, she can hesitate to remove an acknowledged evil? Indeed, it cannot be that England still holds to this evil business, earning the hatred of the officials and people of China, and making herself a reproach among the nations, because she would lose a little revenue were she to forfeit the cultivation of the poppy!

'The writers hope that His Excellency will memorialize his Government to give orders in India and elsewhere to substitute the cultivation of cereals or cotton. Were both nations to rigorously prohibit the growth of the poppy, both the traffic in and the consumption of opium might alike be put an end to. To do away with so great an evil would be a great virtue on England's part; she would strengthen friendly relations and make herself illustrious. How delightful to have so great an act transmitted to after ages!

'This matter is injurious to commercial interests in no ordinary degree. If His Excellency the British Minister cannot, before it is too late, arrange a plan for a joint prohibition (of the traffic), then no matter with what devotedness the writers may plead, *they may be unable to cause the people to put aside ill-feeling, and so strengthen friendly relations as to place them for ever beyond fear of disturbance.* Day and night, therefore, the writers give to this matter most earnest thought, and overpowering is the distress and anxiety it occasions them. Having thus presumed to unbosom themselves, they would be honoured by His Excellency's reply.'

After reading the foregoing in the course of his speech on the opium question in the House of Commons, Mr. Henry Richard continued, 'I don't think I ever read a document in which the accents of sincerity are more apparent than they are in this.' It is no wonder that Sir Rutherford Alcock, after receiving it, should have recorded his own opinion in the following strong language :—

'He had no doubt that the abhorrence expressed by the Government and the people of China for opium as destructive to the Chinese nation, was genuine and deep-seated; and that he was also quite convinced that the Chinese Government could, if it pleased, carry out its threat of developing cultivation to any extent. On the other hand, he believed that *so strong was the popular feeling on the subject, that if Britain would give up the opium revenue, and suppress the cultivation in India, the Chinese Government would have no difficulty in suppressing it in China,* except in the Province of Yunnan, where its authority is in abeyance.' —*Papers relating to the Opium Question, Addendum to Appendix* 4.

TESTIMONY OF BRITISH OFFICIALS.

Testimony of Sir Rutherford Alcock

THAT OPIUM IS A SOURCE OF IMPOVERISHMENT AND RUIN.

5738. *Q.* Can the evils, physical, moral, commercial, and political, as respects individuals, families, and the nation at large, of indulgence in this vice be exaggerated?

A. I have no doubt that where there is a great amount of evil there is always a certain danger of exaggeration; but looking to the *universality of the belief among the Chinese, that whenever a man takes to smoking opium it will probably be the impoverishment and ruin of his family,*—a popular feeling which is universal *both among those who are addicted to it,* who always consider themselves as moral criminals, *and amongst those who abstain from it,* and are merely endeavouring to prevent its consumption,—it is difficult not to conclude that what we hear of it is essentially true, *and that it is a source of impoverishment and ruin to families.*

5746. *Q.* A former witness said that the Chinese themselves all admit that *the effects of opium-smoking are bad;* does your experience bear that out as being their opinion?

A. I think it is universal; I think that the men who smoke opium look upon themselves as morally criminal.—Evidence before the House of Commons Committee on East India Finance, 1871.

Sir Rutherford Alcock's Opinion that the Chinese were infinitely better off without the Opium.

5759. *Q.* I do not know whether you can tell us at all whether the state of the country was better in regard to prosperity and comfort, and that sort of thing, before this great consumption of opium?

A. It is very difficult to entertain any doubt on that point; the Chinese before the century were certainly about the most temperate of races; their food was chiefly vegetable food; they had no stimulants except a mild tobacco and tea, and they seem to have been perfectly content with that; for they have always been known as a most industrious race, cultivating their land to the highest degree, and as being hard-working people. They were that before they had this opium; and tea and mild tobacco certainly could not produce the effects that we now see opium produce, and there is nothing in their history to make us think that there was more pestilence or greater morality, or that they were less capable of performing the work of the nation then; and *I must say that my own impression is, that they were infinitely better off without the opium.—Evidence before House of Commons Committee on East India Finance,* 1871.

Testimony of Sir R. Alcock's Chosen Witness.

Sir Rutherford Alcock, at the Society of Arts, in his paper on 'The Opium Trade,' said:—

Although most of the staple arguments and misleading opinions on opium, and its disastrous effects, come from the missionaries in China, whose good faith I do not question, there is no stronger protest against exaggerated and sensational statements on record than has been supplied by one of their number, the late Dr. Medhurst, of whom it has been truly said, he was 'one of the most able, experienced, and zealous missionaries in China.' Opposed in principle to the opium trade in all its aspects, his statements will be readily accepted as unimpeachable evidence.

[What is the testimony of Sir Rutherford's chosen witness, whose statements he thus admits are 'unimpeachable'?]

Dr. Medhurst said:—

Calculating *the shortened lives, the frequent diseases, and the actual starvation which are the results of opium-smoking in China, we may venture* to assert that this pernicious drug annually destroys myriads of individuals. . . . Slavery was not productive of more misery and death than was the opium traffic, nor were Britons more implicated in the former than in the latter.

Those who grow and sell the drug, while they profit by the speculation, would do well to follow the consumer into the haunts of vice, and *mark the wretchedness, poverty, disease, and death which follow the indulgence;* for did they but know the thousandth part of the evils resulting from it, they would not, they could not, continue to engage in the transaction.

It has been told, and it shall be rung in the ears of the British public again and again, that *opium is demoralizing China*, and becomes the greatest barrier to the introduction of Christianity which can be conceived of.

Testimony of Sir Thomas Wade, C.B.

In the correspondence respecting the revision of the Treaty of Tientsin, he said:—

I cannot endorse the opinion of Messrs. Jardine, Matheson, & Co., that 'the use of opium is not a curse, but a comfort and a benefit, to the hardworking Chinese.' As in all cases of sweeping criticism, those who condemn the opium trade may have been guilty of exaggeration. They have been especially mistaken in representing the British Government and people as responsible for the introduction of opium to the knowledge of the Chinese; the Chinese knew it long before we brought them opium from India. But it is impossible to deny that we bring them that quality which, in the south at all events, tempts them the most, and for which they pay dearest. It is to me vain to think otherwise of the use of the drug in China than as of a habit *many times more pernicious, nationally speaking, than the gin and whisky drinking which we deplore at home.* It takes possession more insidiously, and keeps its hold to the full as tenaciously. I know no case of radical cure. *It has insured, in every case within my knowledge, the steady descent, moral and physical, of the smoker,* and it is, so far, a greater mischief than drink, that it does not, by external evidence of its effect, expose its victim to the loss of repute which is the penalty of habitual drunkenness. There is reason to fear that a higher class than used to smoke in Commissioner Lin's day are now taking to the practice.—*China,* No. 5 (1871) (p. 432).

Testimony of C. H. Aitchison, Esq., C.S., C.S.I., LL.D.,

Chief Commissioner of British Burmah,

ON THE MISERY AND RUIN CAUSED BY OPIUM-SMOKING.

The papers now submitted for consideration present a painful picture of the demoralization, misery, and ruin produced among the Burmese by opium-smoking. Responsible officers in all divisions and districts of the province, and natives everywhere, bear testimony to it. To facilitate examination of the evidence on this point, I have thrown some extracts from the reports into an Appendix to this memorandum. These show that, among the Burmans, the habitual use of the drug saps the physical and mental energies, destroys the nerves, emaciates the body, predisposes to disease, induces indolent and filthy habits of life, destroys self-respect, is one of the most fertile sources of misery, destitution, and crime, fills the jails with men of relaxed frame predisposed to dysentery and cholera, prevents the due extension of cultivation and the development of the land revenue, checks the natural growth of the population, and enfeebles the constitution of succeeding generations.—*From Memorandum addressed to the Government of India, 1880, on the Consumption of Opium in British Burmah.*

Testimony of W. N. Pethick, Esq.,

For several years Vice-Consul and interpreter for the American Government at Tientsin, and who has been for a long time interpreter to Li Hung-chang.

I take it for granted that the ill effects, physical and moral, of opium-smoking are known and admitted by intelligent and unprejudiced people; and, notwithstanding the fine-spun theories of various apologists for the habit, it is enough here to refer to the positive condemnatory testimony of *native victims* of the habit, to *all intelligent and respectable Chinese*, to *foreigners who have had much experience in the country*, and to the united opinion of the foreign medical fraternity in China, from the earliest date of foreign intercourse to the present. —*Extract from letter to the United States' Special Commissioners to China.*

Testimony of Alexander Wylie, Esq.,

Agent of the British and Foreign Bible Society, who for twenty years travelled extensively in China.

Any one who has lived half that time among the Chinese can scarcely have a doubt as to the destructive effects of opium, physically, mentally, and morally. . . . Undoubtedly this is one of the greatest evils with which China is affected, and unless some means be found to check the practice, it bids fair to accomplish the utter destruction, morally and physically, of that great empire.

A Recent Testimony.

The Rev. J. W. Brewer, Wesleyan missionary, in a letter from Hankow, dated January 7, 1882, tells of the success attending missionary effort at Teh-ngan, an important prefectural city to the north-west of Hankow, but there, as elsewhere, opium-smoking prevails to a fearful extent. He says:—'What promises to be a great, if not the greatest obstacle to our work, is the ruinous practice of opium-smoking. It is fearfully prevalent. There are, it is said, more than one hundred dens in the city, and every one asked asserted that more than one-half the adult male population smoked. By open and unsparing denunciations of the vice, by earnest exhortations to reform, and by free use of an illustrated anti-opium tract, we did our best to clear ourselves, as Christian missionaries, from all complicity in the accursed traffic with which, as Englishmen, we are, alas! so closely connected.'

TESTIMONIES OF MEDICAL MEN.

W. LOCKHART, ESQ., F.R.C.S.,

ON OPIUM-SMOKING.

I cannot understand how Dr. Birdwood can say that the smoking of opium is a perfectly innocuous indulgence. This is so great a mistake that it cannot be too strongly protested against. Opium-smoking is extremely injurious, and in the large majority of cases is carried to a constantly increasing extent, and consequent increasing injury on the physical condition of the smoker. Opium-smoking is not so great a social evil as spirit-drinking, but it is a very much greater personal evil to the individual himself. I do not think that opium entices people away from spirit-drinking; those who smoke opium are, in my experience, ever ready to use the spirit, more especially when they cannot get opium. I cannot believe that, if Dr. Birdwood knew from long-continued experience of the effects of opium-smoking on the Chinese, and the frightful consequences thereby induced, he would write as he has expressed himself in his letter to the *Times* of 6th December.

TESTIMONY OF THE LATE SIR BENJAMIN BRODIE

ON THE INJURIOUS ACTION OF OPIUM.

However valuable opium may be when employed as an article of medicine, it is impossible for any one who is acquainted with the subject to doubt that the habitual use of it is productive of the most pernicious consequences, destroying the healthy action of the digestive organs, weakening the powers of the mind as well as the body, and rendering the individual who indulges himself in it a worse than useless member of society. I cannot but regard those who promote the use of opium as an article of luxury as inflicting a most serious injury on the human race.—(Signed) B. C. BRODIE.

The above was also signed by twenty-four of the most distinguished members of the London Faculty, as under—Dr. R. Bright, F.R.S.; Dr. P. Latham;

Dr. Chambers, F.R.S.; Mr. R. Listin, F.R.S.; Dr. Ferguson, F.R.S.; Sir C. Locock, Bart.; Sir J. Forbes, F.R.S.; Dr. M'Leod; Dr. Glendinning, F.R.S.; Mr. J. C. Moore; Dr. Gregory; Dr. Paris, F.R.S.; Sir H. Halford, Bart., F.R.S.; Dr. R. T. Thompson; Dr. Hodgkin, F.R.S.; Mr. F. Tynell; Mr. Cesar Hawkins, F.R.S.; Dr. B. Travers, F.R.S.; Sir H. Holland, Bart., F.R.S.; Dr. James Watson, F.R.S.; Mr. Ashton Key; Mr. Antony White; Dr. James Johnston; Dr. J. C. B. Williams, F.R.S.

The 'Lancet' on Opium-Smoking, and on the Views put forth by Sir George Birdwood and Surgeon-General Moore.

His [Sir George Birdwood's] view of the question is deprived of much of the weight which his Indian experience would give it by the frank admission that his opinion was formed when a student in Edinburgh, before he went to India at all; while his extraordinary denial that the smoke of opium possesses any narcotic influence, because the constituents of opium are not volatilizable, will raise a suspicion of the value of his other assertions. . . . It will not be easy to convince the medical profession that either individuals or races are benefited by the habitual use of a stimulant which notoriously, in its moderate use, becomes a greater necessity than does the moderate use of alcohol. The opium-eater, after a very brief habituation, is wretched and feeble without his artificial strength, and the moderate employment of opium is comparable rather to what is now regarded as the habitually excessive use of alcohol than to its really moderate use. The moderate and even the minimum opium-eater is a slave to his stimulant as the moderate alcohol-drinker is not. The testimony on this point is overwhelming, and so also is the evidence of the rapidity with which the opium-eater becomes enslaved, and the extreme difficulty and rarity of rescue. The mass of evidence on this point—as an example of which we may mention the Chinese consular reports lately referred to in these columns—is altogether ignored by Mr. Moore, and *à fortiori* by Sir George Birdwood, the former contenting himself with a covert sneer at the statements of missionaries (who have probably enjoyed better opportunities for observation than any one else), and by the assertion and demonstration of the fact that recovery from the opium habit is a *possible* thing, which no one dreamed of denying. It is, moreover, difficult to attach much weight to any opinion of a writer who at one page admits that 'confessedly the practice of using opium, in common with indulgence in alcohol, exerts sufficiently deleterious influences,' and at another asserts that 'the moderate use of opium is, under innumerable circumstances, beneficial to mankind both in health and sickness,' and who deliberately defends as harmless the habitual administration of opium to young children.

Excuse 2.—THE CHINESE NOT SINCERE IN THEIR DESIRE TO SUPPRESS OPIUM.

On this point the testimony is overwhelming, but the following may suffice.

TESTIMONY OF SIR RUTHERFORD ALCOCK.

Before the House of Commons Committee on East India Finance, in 1871, he gave evidence as under:—

5808. *Q.* You have told us that the Chinese Government have a most lively feeling of the enormous evils attending the import of opium, and the consumption of opium in their country; and that you believe they are *sincerely* desirous of *not only doing away with the growth of opium* in their own country, but also *of preventing the import of it from foreign countries?*

A. Yes.

5740. *Q.* I think I understood you, in reply to my honourable friend, to say that you believed that the *Chinese Government were perfectly sincere* in their desire to put an end to the consumption of opium?

A. I believe they are.

5725. *A.* I have estimated the absolute interest of the Chinese Government in the Indian trade at about a million and a half sterling; and in reference to this I may mention that not only in the conference that took place with the ministers of the Tsung-li Yamên, a minute of which I read at the last meeting of the Committee, but also at different times, officially or privately, *they have shown the greatest readiness to give up the whole revenue if they could only induce the British Government to co-operate with them in any way to put it down.* My own conviction is firm, that whatever degree of honesty may be attributed to the officials and to the central Government, there is that at work in their minds *that they would not hesitate one moment to-morrow if they could to enter into any arrangement with the British Government, and say, 'Let our revenue go; we care nothing about it. What we want is to stop the consumption of opium, which we conceive is impoverishing the country, and demoralizing and brutalizing our people.'*

5884. *Q.* But I understand, from your evidence, that you consider *that they are thoroughly in earnest* in the matter, and that they are only prevented from doing anything by the superior power of England in forcing the sale?

A. That is the general tendency of my evidence, that they are honest in so far as they really desire, or would desire, to see the consumption of opium put a stop to, and that they feel that they are powerless in face of the determination of England to have it inserted in the tariff.

Testimony of Li Hung-Chang.

The following very important letter, written by His Excellency the Grand Secretary and Viceroy Li, in answer to one addressed to him on the opium question by the secretary of the Society for the Suppression of the Opium Trade, deserves, and should have, the thoughtful attention of the people of England. The influential position of the writer, who may, perhaps, be briefly described as the Gladstone of China, gives importance to his letter, which it is impossible to read without feelings of humiliation and shame. This distinguished man says :—
'Opium is a subject in the discussion of which England and China can never meet on common ground. China views the whole question from a moral standpoint; England from a fiscal. England would sustain a source of revenue in India, while China contends for the lives and prosperity of her people.'

These are remarkable words. Are they true? Let a Minister of the British Crown answer the question. The Marquis of Hartington, speaking in his place in the House of Commons, said :—

'It is not my intention on this occasion to assent to any resolution, or to say anything which would have any tendency to disturb, to endanger, or even to diminish so important a branch of Indian revenue as that derived from the opium trade. . . . I must make some protest against the invitation . . . . . to consider this question from the point of view of the dictates of morality, as they are entertained by some members of this House, and to altogether neglect the subject as it relates to India and Indian policy. My hon. friend says he should be sorry to be suspected of judging this question on the low standard of Indian finance. But it is a question of Indian finance.'

LETTER FROM HIS EXCELLENCY THE GRAND SECRETARY AND VICEROY LI.

'Viceroy's Yamen, Tien-tsin, China,
May 24th, 1881.

'Sir,—It gave me great pleasure to receive your letter, dated February 25th, with its several enclosures, sent on behalf of the Anglo-Oriental Society for the Suppression of the Opium Trade.

'Your society has long been known to me and many of my countrymen, and I am sure that all—save victims to the opium habit, and those who have not a spark of right feeling—would unite with me in expressing a sense of gratitude for the philanthropic motives and efforts of the society in behalf of China.

'To know that so many of your countrymen have united to continually protest against the evils of the opium traffic, and thus second the efforts China has long been making to free herself from this curse, is a source of great satisfaction to my Government, to whom I have communicated a copy of your letter. The sense of injury which China has so long borne with reference to opium finds some relief in the sympathy which a society like yours existing in England bespeaks.

'*Opium is a subject in the discussion of which England and China can never meet on common ground. China views the whole question from a moral standpoint; England from a fiscal. England would sustain a source of revenue in India, while China contends for the lives and prosperity of her people. The ruling motive with China is to repress opium by heavy taxation everywhere, whereas with England the manifest object is to make opium cheaper, and thus increase and stimulate the demand in China.*

'With motives and principles so radically opposite, it is not surprising that the discussion commenced at Chefoo in 1876 has up to the present time been fruitless of good results. The whole record of this discussion shows that inducement and persuasion have been used in behalf of England to prevent any additional taxation of opium in China, and objections made to China exercising her undoubted right to regulate her own taxes—at least with regard to opium.

'I may take the opportunity to assert here, once for all, that the single aim of my Government in taxing opium will be in the future, as it has always been in the past, to repress the traffic—never the desire to gain revenue from such a source. Having failed to kill a serpent, who would be so rash as to nurse it in his bosom? *If it be thought that China countenances the import for the revenue it brings, it should be known that my Government will gladly cut off all such revenue in order to stop the import of opium. My sovereign has never desired his empire to thrive upon the lives or infirmities of his subjects.*

'In discussing opium taxation, a strange concern, approaching to alarm, has been shown in behalf of China, lest she should sacrifice her revenue; and yet objection and protest are made against rates which could be fixed for collection at the ports and in the interior. The Indian Government is in the background at every official discussion of the opium traffic, and every proposed arrangement must be forced into a shape acceptable to that Government and harmless to its revenues. This is not as it should be. Each Government should be left free to deal with opium according to its own lights. If China, out of compassion for her people, wishes to impose heavy taxes to discountenance and repress the use of opium, the Indian Government should be equally free, if it see fit, to preserve its revenue by increasing the price of its opium as the demand for it diminishes in China.

'The poppy is certainly surreptitiously grown in some parts of China, notwithstanding the laws and frequent Imperial edicts prohibiting its cultivation. Yet this unlawful cultivation no more shows that the Government approves of it than other crimes committed in the empire by lawless subjects indicate approval by the Government of such crimes. In like manner, the present import duty on opium was established, not from choice, but because China submitted to the adverse decision of arms. *The war must be considered as China's standing protest against legalizing such a revenue.*

'My Government is impressed with the necessity of making strenuous efforts to control this flood of opium before it overwhelms the whole country. The new treaty with the United States, containing the prohibitory clause against opium, encourages the belief that the broad principles of justice and feelings of humanity will prevail in future relations between China and Western nations. My Government will take effective measures to enforce the laws against the cultivation of the poppy in China, and otherwise check the use of opium; and *I earnestly hope that your society and all right-minded men of your country will support the efforts China is now making to escape from the thraldom of opium.*—I am, Sir, your obedient servant,

'Li Hung-chang.

'To F. Storrs Turner, Esq., Secretary to the Anglo-Oriental Society for the Suppression of the Opium Trade, London.'

Popular Feeling against Opium shown by the Honour paid to the Man who tried to keep Opium out of China.

It is a fact that those mandarins who have been the most hostile to the trade, and have done most to put it down, have been the most popular men in China. I might refer to many; let one suffice as the most noted of all—the Grand Commissioner Lin—the man who shut up our merchants and deprived them of their dinners till they gave up opium, which he destroyed with his own hand, to the value of £2,000,000—the man who so effectually shut opium out of China, that neither rich nor poor could get their supply till the navies of England came to their relief. That man was loved and honoured more than any modern statesman in China, and to this day they celebrate his praises and bless his memory. So much was he honoured in Canton, that when he was driven out by English influence, and disgraced by the Emperor to please us, the whole of Canton rose to do him honour; and as he was borne by the citizens through their streets, they made him change his boots at each gate, and, according to Chinese fashion, hung up the old ones as trophies of a good man, and as a hint to the man who stepped into his shoes to walk in his steps. If any man doubts this fact, let him go to Canton and look at Lin's boots.—*Rev. James Johnston, formerly missionary to China, now minister of St. James's Free Church, Glasgow.*

Popular Feeling in China against Opium-Smoking shown by the General Distrust of Opium-Smokers.

It is well known to all in China that this popular feeling against the use of opium manifests itself in a thousand ways; for example, a man who is known to take opium to the smallest extent has difficulty in getting credit; his countrymen cannot trust him. A respectable parent will never give his daughter in marriage to an opium-smoker, and from the day a man takes to the opium pipe he becomes an object of distrust, or pity, or dislike; and so strong is the feeling of distrust, and the dread of the ultimate issue of this vicious habit, that every Christian Church that is known in China makes it an invariable rule that no man who smokes opium shall ever be admitted as a member. And this rule is found necessary, not only because of the foreign estimate of the habit, but because the moral tone of the people of China would be justly offended at the toleration of the vice.—'*The Opium Trade in China,*' *by Rev. James Johnston* (published 1858).

THE GROWTH OF OPIUM IN CHINA NO PROOF OF INSINCERITY.

Testimony of Sir Rutherford Alcock.

In reference to the growth of opium in China, in his evidence before the House of Commons Committee in 1871, he said:—

5696. I think it will be seen the substance of the whole is this: that there is a very large and increasing cultivation of the poppy in

China, that the Chinese Government are seriously contemplating, if they cannot come to any terms or arrangement with the British Government for restricting the area of growth in India, and either gradually or suddenly putting an end to its importation, as they think

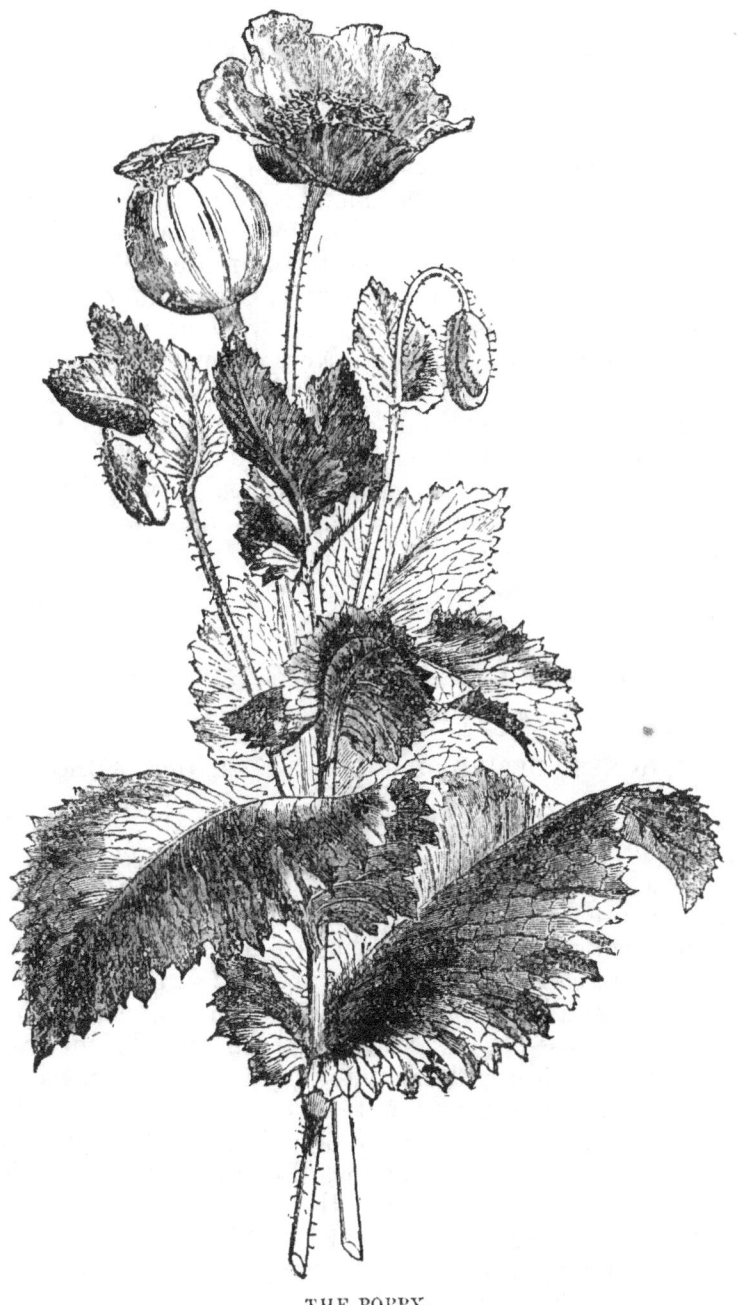

THE POPPY.

they have the power to do, the cultivation without stint in China, and producing opium at a much cheaper rate. Having done that, they think they will afterwards be able to stamp out the opium produce among themselves. I doubt their power to do so, but that is their theory.

TESTIMONY OF W. N. PETHICK, ESQ.,

For several years Vice-Consul and interpreter for the American Government at Tientsin, and who has been for a long time interpreter to Li Hung-chang, in a long letter to the U.S. Special Commissioners to China, congratulating them on the treaty they had concluded with China,

ON THE GENUINE DESIRE OF CHINA TO SUPPRESS OPIUM.

It is a mistake to say that since the opium war with England, in 1842, the Chinese Government has never shown a genuine desire to limit or suppress the opium traffic. The printed laws of the empire, imperial edict, memorials from members of the Government at Peking, and from provincial authorities, and remarks by ministers of the Chinese Foreign Office addressed to the representatives of foreign Governments, in documents and in conversation, fully attest the fact that China has never consented to bear without murmur the great wrong which was forced upon her. Nor, because imperial edicts are set at naught, and the cultivation of the poppy commissioned by officials in some parts of the country, is it fair to tax the Government of China with indifference to the spread of the evil. *Blood and treasure were spent freely in combating its introduction, and, though defeated in war, the Government has not remained a silent and unfeeling witness of this blight extending over the country. The public archives down to the present time bear witness to the fact.*

TESTIMONY OF REV. J. HUDSON TAYLOR, M.R.C.S.,

Founder of the China Inland Mission,

ON THE HONEST DESIRE OF CHINA TO STOP OPIUM-SMOKING.

To our mind, nothing is more clear than that the Chinese had both *the right, the power, and the will to stamp out the use of opium in China* at the time when they first came into collision with the power of England. We are fully convinced that but for England they would then have accomplished this; and hence we feel that *England is morally responsible for every ounce of opium* NOW *produced in China*, as well as for that imported from abroad. This, it seems to us, cannot be too clearly asserted and recognised. . . . Now, to stamp out the vice would be no easy matter, even were China unfettered. We are persuaded that China has the honest *desire* to put an end to the vice, and we feel assured that she has the full *intention* of doing so. The present toleration of the growth of native opium is, in our judgment as in hers, her only resource. She wishes to make the importation of Indian opium unprofitable, for England's *profession* of Christian principle she too fully believes to be hollow and insincere to longer entertain any hope from it on the score of either justice or mercy. But if the import trade can be made unprofitable, or sufficiently precarious to induce England to withdraw her pressure, China knows herself to be well able first to circumscribe, and then to abolish, the home production. Bad as things now are, and worse as they are becoming, we have not a doubt that she could so far stamp opium-smoking out in a generation, that it would no longer be an extensive national vice.—*China's Millions, April* 1882.

DAVID M'LAREN, ESQ., J.P., D.L. (EDINBURGH),
At a meeting at the Society of Arts, said:—

With what grace could the Chinese prevent their own people growing poppies if at the same time they received opium from India? Here is a governor, who has on the one side a native grower of poppy, and on the other a foreign vendor of opium; how can he prohibit the former while obliged to tolerate the latter?—*Journal of Society of Arts*, p. 232.

THE HON. SIR EDWARD FRY,
One of the judges of the High Court of Justice, writes thus concerning the growth of opium in China:—

But then it is said, 'Oh, that would be all very well if the resistance of China to opium were an honest one; but it is not an honest one, it is only a sham, and we have proof positive that it is only a sham, for China herself permits, nay encourages, the growth of opium.' Now, it is perfectly true that China, which used to punish the growth of the poppy with death, has within the last few years connived at, or, if you will, permitted and encouraged its growth; but it is equally clear to my mind that this policy has been dictated, not by any willingness to allow the use of opium, but simply by the feeling that, as its consumption is inevitable through the pressure of England, it is better that the opium to be consumed should be raised in China than in India. 'If we must see our people use the accursed drug, let us, and not England, gain the profit, and let us defeat England's selfish policy, and at least taste the sweets of revenge.'

I believe, therefore, not only that the sentiment of China remains true in its hatred of opium, but that we English, by the policy which we have pursued, are morally responsible for every acre of land in China which is withdrawn from the cultivation of grain and devoted to that of the poppy; so that the fact of the growth of the drug in China ought only to increase our sense of responsibility.—*England, China, and Opium*, p. 16.

Excuse 3.—'THE BRITISH GOVERNMENT HAS NOT FORCED CHINA TO ADMIT OPIUM.'

That England has forced China to admit opium is shown by the following:—

TESTIMONY OF SIR RUTHERFORD ALCOCK, K.C.B.

5809. *Q.* Now, is there anything in our treaties *to force them* to take our opium?
A. Yes, it is put in the tariff of articles of import.

5810. *Q.* Then they are bound to allow the free import of opium?
A. That was the condition introduced into the treaty which Lord Elgin made.

5811. *Q.* But we do not enforce the purchase?

A. Not the purchase; but they cannot prohibit the import of opium; it is amongst the admitted articles on the tariff.

5812. *Q.* Then, notwithstanding that the Chinese Government are so sensible of the demoralization of their people caused by the import of opium, they cannot prevent our sending it there,—*we force them by treaty to take it from us?*

A. That is so, in effect.

5813. *Q.* We have *forced* the Government to enter into a treaty to allow their subjects to take it?

A. Yes, precisely.

5814. *Q.* Is it any wonder that the Chinese Government complain of our conduct in that respect?

A. No, I do not think it is any wonder.

5815. *Q.* What should we say if the Chinese imposed the like restrictions upon us?

A. I think that our answer to them for putting it into the treaty is, 'You cannot prevent it being smuggled, and the lesser evil is to admit it as a legitimate article of trade.'

5816. *Q.* But is it not for them to judge of that, and not for us?

A. No doubt, if two nations are negotiating together on equal terms, each should have a voice.

5865. *Q.* But suppose the Chinese Government were to say, 'We decline to admit opium; we will not renew the treaty except on the condition of excluding opium altogether?'

A. I think they could only do that on the same principle as that on which Prince Gortchakoff declared that Russia would not submit to the continued neutralization of the Black Sea,—*they must be prepared to fight for it.*

5876. *Q.* As I understand you, you say that the Chinese have made a treaty from which it is not possible for them to escape?

A. It is not possible for them to escape from it except by a declaration that they will not submit to what they conceive to be injurious terms.

5877. *Q.* The only way that they can escape from it is by a war?

A. A war, or a declaration that they are ready to go to war rather than submit any longer.—*Evidence before the House of Commons Committee on East India Finance,* 1871.

Testimony of Commissioner Kwei-lang.

The Chinese Commissioner Kwei-lang, pleading with Lord Elgin, in October 1858, for some forbearance as to carrying into execution certain of the articles of the Treaty of Tientsin, wrote as follows:—

'When the Chinese Commissioners negotiated a treaty with your Excellency at Tientsin, British vessels of war were lying in that port; there was a pressure of an armed force, a state of excitement and alarm, and the treaty had to be signed at once without a moment's delay. Deliberation was out of the question; the Commissioners had no alternative but to accept the conditions forced upon them.'

—*Correspondence relative to Lord Elgin's Mission,* pp. 408–9.

Testimony of Sir Thomas Wade.

Nothing that has been gained, it must be remembered, was received from the free-will of the Chinese; more, the concessions made to us have been, from first to last, extorted against the conscience of the nation—in defiance, that is to say, of the moral convictions of its educated men—not merely of the office-holders, whom we call mandarins, and who are numerically but a small proportion of the educated class, but of the millions who are saturated with a knowledge of the history and philosophy of their country. — *China, No. 5. (1871). Correspondence respecting the Revision of the Treaty of Tientsin. Memorandum by Mr. Wade (now Sir Thomas Wade, K.C.B., British Minister at Pekin)* (p. 432).

Testimony of Lord Elgin.

The concessions obtained in the treaty from the Chinese Government are not in themselves extravagant, but in the eyes of the Chinese Government they amount to a revolution. *They have been extorted, therefore, from its fears.*—Blue Book, p. 348.

Testimony of Rev. H. Grattan Guinness.

We English send the Chinese thousands of tons of opium; we send them more of opium than of anything else; we have long sent it to them; we send it to them though we see the fearful ravages resulting from its use; we send it to them though their Government protests against it, though their Government has not ceased to protest against our conduct in doing so for the last seventy-seven years. For forty-five years we smuggled it into their country by means of armed vessels manned by desperadoes; and when, stung to passionate resistance by the wicked and daring conduct of our smugglers, they rose against us and resolved to put a stop to this nefarious traffic at all costs, we sent our men-of-war up their rivers, burned their junks, destroyed their forts, slaughtered their soldiers, scattered their forces, and compelled them to permit the continuance of our commerce, the main export of which was opium, and to pay the expenses of the war which our unrighteousness had provoked. Nor did we stop here; unsatisfied that this most profitable trade should exist merely by Chinese sufferance, we took the opportunity, which a later war and later victories over them afforded, to oblige their Government to legalize the hated traffic. Since that act, our conduct, though branded as immoral by every section of their people, has had the sanction of the letter of their law; since then the trade has flourished more than ever; opium ships and tea ships moor unmolested side by side; Indian opium pours into China without resistance; and China herself, despairing at length of all power to prevent its introduction, permits the poison-bearing plant to be cultivated in its midst, and meditates, though with intense reluctance, such an increase of the home-grown article as will at least arrest the outflow of some millions of money which they now annually pay us in exchange for the fatal foreign drug.

Testimony of Sir Edward Fry.

One of the most important results of that treaty [the Treaty of Tientsin] was that by the agreement of 8th November 1858, made in pursuance of this treaty, the Chinese Government *yielded to our pressure*, and admitted opium as an article of import subject to a certain duty. The whole history of the trade, and the provisions with which the concession was surrounded, all show that in this concession the Chinese *yielded only to superior force*. Such a course of violence seems to me wicked in the last degree. I believe, but I will not now urge, that opium is a poison, and that it ruins the bodies and souls of thousands of men. For my line of thought no such proposition is needful; it is enough that the Chinese Government honestly objected to it. But I will carry my argument a step further, and without discussing whether some men can eat opium without harm, or whether it acts first on the mind or the body, or whether it is worse than gin or not so bad; this I will say, almost without fear of contradiction, that opium is a drug of such a character that the Chinese Government were at liberty, if they so determined, to hold it to be a poison, and that the Indian Government and English diplomacy had no right to say, 'You shall not hold it as a poison.' . . . .

Many people will be convinced by such facts as these, that the desire of the Chinese Government to exclude opium was and is a sound one; but whether this be so or not, no one who affects to be a reasonable creature can say that their objection to opium was frivolous; no man can say that their fixed opinion on the point was or is unreasonable. Even if it were frivolous and unreasonable, it is at least doubtful to my mind whether any foreign country had a right by force to overrule such a decision of a Government, and thereby to cripple the authority of the state, and to help on anarchy; but, being neither frivolous nor unreasonable, I say that such a decision ought to have been respected, and that its being *overborne by force was an act of high-handed injustice*, for which we can feel nothing but shame. . . .

No picture can be more shocking than that of one nation *forcing* on another a drug which the weaker one believes, and believes with a dreadful truth, to be a most horrible curse.

Why does not China crush the Opium Trade?

It seems scarcely credible that England could be guilty of such a crime as this! [giving the shelter of the British flag to opium vessels. This was written before the trade in opium was legalized.] But facts, sad facts, are these. England has done worse than this. She has not only employed her skill and commerce to tempt, and seduce, and ruin the people of China; she has employed the terror of her name, and the protection of her flag, to keep these opium vessels anchored within sight of the helpless slaves of a vice which she has created,—she holds the cup to their lip, and dares them to cast it away. When she says that she does not compel them to drink, it is a mockery alike to justice and humanity. China, if left to herself, would long ere this have banished this trade in opium. Numerous though the smokers are, they are but a mere fraction of her vast population—the former are counted by millions, the latter by hundreds of millions; and, *as an empire, China has shown a steady and consistent hostility to the trade.* You may say, *Why then not drive these vessels from her shores and crush the trade*, seeing it is against her laws? I can but reply—*China did so once, and it cost her life's blood.* In 1839 she dashed the cup from her lips, England took up the broken fragments, put them together, and compelled her to fill that cup with the blood of her best citizens, and six millions sterling of her pure silver. Can we wonder that China is afraid to touch English opium or the English flag again?—*Rev. James Johnston.*

Excuse 4.—'IF OPIUM WAS FORCED UPON CHINA, WE ARE NOT RESPONSIBLE FOR WHAT WAS DONE BY OTHERS LONG AGO.'

But we are responsible for *continuing to force opium upon China*, and under solemn obligation to put an end to our national connection with the dreadful business. This point has been put very clearly by

Mr. Justice Fry.

'But what,' it will be said, 'is the use of going back to the history of our relations with China long years ago, and to the doings of a generation that has nearly passed away? Why trouble about the irrevocable past? The thing is done and ended, and the sin, if sin there were, is accomplished; but it was the sin not of us, but of our fathers.' The answer is a very plain one. The thing is not done and ended; the policy which our fathers pursued we are pursuing still. *The resistance to the introduction of opium, which led to the Opium War, is still made with a noble persistency by the Chinese authorities and the Chinese people, and we are, with a yet greater but most ignoble persistency, forcing the accursed thing into the ports and up the rivers of China.* The wicked policy of thus violating the national conscience of China rests on our shoulders, as a burden not of past but of present sin; our fathers slew the prophets, and we build their sepulchres.—*England, China, and Opium*, p. 13.

We are Responsible.

You may, perhaps, truly say that, thus far, you have been altogether innocent in this matter—that you have had no part in these iniquities; that you never knew—that you never suspected—that such a traffic was carried on by your fellow-countrymen, and under the British flag. But this you can no longer say. The case is altered *now*. From this time forth, if you do not protest against these iniquities—if you do not endeavour, according to your ability, to put them down—you become, in your measure, a partaker of them, and (by your careless connivance) a tacit accomplice in the crimes of your fellow-countrymen.

He who stands by unconcerned while murder is committed, and (still more) he who shelters the murderer and facilitates his escape, according to all law, divine and human, is justly deemed an accomplice in the crime. What, then, shall be said of you—what will you in your conscience judge concerning yourself—if you (now knowing the fact that the opium trade is every year destroying thousands and tens of thousands of the people of China) shall go on unconcerned and reckless, without lifting up either your voice or your hand to protest against or prevent such wholesale murder?—*Iniquities of the Opium Trade in China*, by the Rev. A. S. Thelwall, M.A.

Our Duty.

Even if China be insincere, even if she should, in case of our ceasing to force opium on her, fill the whole void by the home-grown drug, our duty is still clear—we ought still to cleanse our hands from the vile trade. But if, as I believe is the case, we are forcing our opium on an unwilling Government, and are doing all in our power to ruin her people, and to frustrate her efforts to benefit them, then our national sin is of yet deeper dye, then the call to exertion on the part of those who oppose the trade is louder and clearer still.—*Sir Edward Fry.*

Excuse 5.—'IF WE DO NOT SEND OPIUM TO CHINA, OTHERS WILL.'

We are considering, for once, a moral question; and to say that some one else would do a wrong if I did not, is no excuse for me. Brown murdered Smith for £1000 of blood money; he alleges, as a sufficient excuse, that if he had not done so, Robinson would have murdered the unfortunate man, or even that Smith would have murdered himself; and that in either of these events he, Brown, would have lost his £1000. From a financial point of view, Brown's reasoning is admirable. But can any man suppose such a defence good in any form whatsoever, whether of law or of conscience? It is precisely the old argument that was used with regard to the slave trade, and was exposed with so much humour by Cowper,—

> 'Besides, if we do, the French, Dutch, and Danes
> Will heartily thank us, no doubt, for our pains:
> If we do not buy the poor creatures, they will:
> And tortures and groans will be multiplied still.'

—*England, Opium, and China*, by Sir Edward Fry, p. 42.

Excuse 6.—'THAT OPIUM-SMOKING IN CHINA IS NOT WORSE THAN INTOXICATING DRINK IN ENGLAND.'

Opium no worse than Alcohol.

We are often told, in this House and elsewhere, that though, no doubt, opium-smoking is a great evil, it is not worse than the gin and whisky drinking that prevails among ourselves. Well, it need not be worse, and yet be bad enough. But what a strange argument to be used by a Christian nation, to say: 'There is a habit among ourselves which, according to the concurrent testimony of ministers of religion, magistrates, judges, medical men,—of all who are concerned in the administration of the law, or who are caring for the health and morals of the people,—is the most prolific source of disease, crime, and misery, and what we force on the Chinese is not much worse than that; and what right have they to complain?'—*Speech of Mr. Henry Richard, M.P.*

THE OPIUM MONOPOLY.

A PROPOSAL; VERY CANDID, IF NOT VERY WISE.

A very remarkable article on the Opium Monopoly appeared in *The Friend of India and Statesman*, published in Calcutta, June 25, 1881. Let Englishmen read and ponder the following delightfully candid extracts:—

MORAL SCRUPLES v. £7,000,000.

'No one has anything to gain by doing away with the opium revenue, except in the form of the satisfaction of conscientious feeling. It is hard to believe that any moral scruple could in the scale weigh down seven millions sterling a year, that the indulgence of any sentiment could be purchased at such a price. . . . It seems hardly possible that we should at any time be compelled to increase so many bad taxes in order to repeal a single impost, which does no harm in this country, whatever may be its effects in China.

THE OPIUM AGITATION NOT TO BE DESPISED.

'It is, however, by no means wise to despise the present opium agitation in England, as if it could not possibly lead to anything. We must remember that the motive at work is precisely the same as that which animated the anti-slavery movement, and that England did in fact pay twenty millions sterling as compensation to West India planters for the loss of their slaves. . . . The proper lesson of the anti-slavery movement is that a mere moral sentiment, when it is strongly enforced by public orators, may be strong enough to move the English masses to consent to, or rather to compel, the sacrifice of enormous sums of money; but it is by no means certain that if the opium revenue were abolished, England would pay anything. . . . The sacrifice of other people's money on a scale, however large, is one that a nation will make readily enough at the bidding of conscience. *If a certain number of electors joined the movement, so as to make it worth a hundred votes or so to each candidate at a Parliamentary election, the thing would be done.* Both candidates would take the pledge to avoid loss, and both parties would give in their adherence. There can be little doubt that even now some votes are to be gained in some places by attacking the opium monopoly, and none can be got anywhere by defending it. Such considerations will now-a-days have greater weight than any number of despatches from a Governor-General in Council. We should say that the opium revenue must now be pronounced in danger, and that those interested in its defence, that is to say, all Indian taxpayers, should look to it.

TIME TO SET OUR HOUSE IN ORDER.

'It is, indeed, time that our house should be set in order. The objections to the opium revenue which really tell with the average English voter, who is the master of the situation and of the country, are not essential to the raising of the revenue, and may, if our action be not too long delayed, be removed in time to save the exchequer from ruinous loss. . . . The opium trade may be defensible, but it is hardly a business in which the Governor-General should take part in his official capacity. If he must touch it, we should recommend that the contact should not be too close. The officers of the opium department are an excellent set of men, who, in spite of their theory that the drug is most useful, never consume any of it themselves; but it is not a pleasant spectacle to see them moving about the country, tempting cultivators with advances on the part of Government to grow the poppy, or to watch them at some station receiving the juice from thousands of clients. The Government godowns at Patna are most interesting, but those who watch the process by which the drug is made into cakes for India and balls for China, may fairly doubt if this is a business which should be performed by Government servants. An opium auction is one of the sights of Calcutta; it is seldom that one can see property worth a million sterling change hands in half an hour, at rates which rise and fall even during the sale itself in a manner which awakens the keenest spirit of gambling; but is it quite consistent with our ideas that a Government secretary should preside once a month at such an auction of such an article on the account of the state? The retail sale of the drug at Government treasuries, a cake at a time, will to many seem still more anomalous. Government will not sell a bottle of gin or brandy; why, then, a cake of opium? . . .

THE MONEY WITHOUT THE ODIUM.

'If the monopoly were abandoned, Government would still control the cultivation, by system of permits, as in the case of *ganja*. . . . There are many traders who would undertake the work of manufacture, employing the present staff if necessary. And there would be no lack of competition for the business of storing the drug in Calcutta, or of selling it to the exporters. It may be confidently anticipated that the business would be better done in every respect by persons whose success as traders depended on it, than by the salaried officers now employed. . . . The duty levied would be proportionate to the average profit to Government on each chest under the present system, and the amount of the receipts would depend on the quantity manufactured. If private enterprise was successful, the demand would increase, and the revenue would gain; in the unlikely event of its failure to obtain as good results as the direct action of Government, there would be a falling off. But whether it is more or less than it is now, the opium revenue would be comparatively secure. It would be hardly open to attack simply as a tax on a pernicious drug. The Marquis of Hartington and the Liberal Government at home have pledged themselves to try to effect some such change, and if the Bengal Government is well advised, it will not interpose the helpless objection, *non possumus*.'

Let not Lord Hartington or the Government think that the people of England will be hoodwinked by the abolition of the monopoly, if the abolition is only to be a prelude to the transfer of the wretched business to private enterprise, and the maintenance of the revenue in another form.

It is too late to attempt to fool the country by any such device. Nothing less is demanded than that the Government of China shall be absolutely free to admit or not to admit opium, as in the interests of the people of China it may be thought expedient. This is plainly stated, as under, in the memorial to Mr. Gladstone :—

'Suggestions have been made of some scheme by which, instead of the Government being itself the manufacturers and dealers in the drug, encouragement would be given to private persons to assume such a position, and the Government would, by means of a licence or some other form of taxation, endeavour to *keep its present revenue*, and to *get rid of the odium* which attaches to the trade. Such a scheme, if it should ever be adopted, would involve a continuation of that pressure on the Chinese which is the most odious part of our present system, and *would not lessen by a feather's weight the burden of our present sin, but rather add to it the fresh stain of hypocrisy*. It cannot be forgotten that, speaking generally, we are not dealing with a trade which requires to be checked, but with a monopoly, which ceases the moment it is not exercised; that the Indian Government is a despotism, and that in a despotism to permit is to do; and that to hand over to private individuals a trade which we have created and increased by wrong, and could immediately extinguish, would be a mere piece of moral legerdemain. *Nothing short of an actual withdrawal from all complicity in the trade, and of a real and zealous co-operation with the Chinese Government, could satisfy the exigencies of conscience.'—From 'Memorial' to Mr. Gladstone.*—For signatures to this memorial, see pp. 109, 110.

A Larger Revenue with Less Labour.

It might fairly be expected in this instance, as in most others, that private enterprise would increase and cheapen production, *and that an excise duty would give Government a larger revenue*, with infinitely less labour and expense in administrative machinery than is at present incurred.—*'How India is Governed,' by Alex. Mackenzie, late member of the Legislative Council, Madras.*

An Erroneous Issue.

It has by some persons been suggested as a remedy, that England should abandon the monopoly practically in favour of private trade. This is a strangely erroneous issue to raise; for surely it is absolutely unimportant whether we raise revenue by a monopoly or by a tax. To me it seems idle, or very nearly idle, to harp on the difference between the Indian Government growing opium and permitting it to be grown; for the responsibilities of a despotic government are greater than those of a free state. . . .

But what I do object to is that, being interested, as I have pointed out, in the sale of opium, the Government has worked both tax and monopoly alike for one purpose, and for one purpose only, viz. the acquisition of the largest amount of gain, and that without regard to the moral results on China, and in defiance of the wishes of the Governmen and people of China.—*Mr. Justice Fry in 'England, China, and Opium.'*

THE OPIUM TRADE AND BRITISH COMMERCE.

The Opium Trade with China Injurious to British Commerce.

Extracts from *An Inquiry into the Results of the Opium Trade with China, including its bearing on the Export of British Manufactures*, by DAVID M'LAREN, Esq., J.P.

Our commerce with China has been the most disappointing chapter in the history of free trade. It has resulted, whatever be the cause, in a state of matters utterly anomalous.

[Mr. M'Laren then goes into detail, and after giving the total amounts for certain years of the imports from China, and exports to China, and showing how small a proportion of our export trade is done with China, he says:—]

But striking as these figures are, the full force of the contrast is not sufficiently brought out, unless we also remember that the empire, where we are so unsuccessful in our commerce, contains much more than a third of the population of the globe,—and that population intensely mercantile in its character,—and that it is intersected by innumerable canals, affording the cheapest means of conveyance from the coast to the interior; while India, with one or two exceptions, has scarcely a road or canal worthy of the name. Yet to 'this magnificent market,' as the committee call it, we send much the same quantity of goods that we do to Egypt, to such petty republics as La Plata or Chili, or the slave population of Cuba!

Table of British Exports, on the average of 4 years, ending 1857, *to*
Egypt, with a population of   4,000,000,   £1,548,674
Cuba and St. Domingo, with a population of 2,400,000,   1,734,448
Chili, with a population of   1,400,000,   1,417,314
China, with a population of   400,000,000,   1,736,191

Were the amount of the opium trade converted into British manufactures, the shipments to China, instead of barely equalling those to some of the petty States already named, would amount to the whole of them together, and of several more besides, and would place it next to the United States as our best customer.

'Cease sending us so much opium,' said the chief magistrate of Shanghai, 'and we shall be enabled to take your manufactures.'

[Other tables are then given, and Mr. M'Laren proceeds:—]

For twelve or thirteen years after the opening of the India and China trade of 1813, opium formed scarcely one-half of the exports to China. In 1858, cotton was £393,493, and opium £8,241,032, or *ninety per cent.* of the whole!

It is impossible to resist the conclusion to be drawn from these tables. If the Chinese take value for their exports in one form, they cannot at the same time take it in another; and further, as will be seen shortly, the more they take in opium, the more they diminish their productive power, and subsequent ability to become profitable customers in any trade. The commercial part of our inquiry cannot be better summed up than in the words of Captain Elliot, British superintendent of trade in China: the opium traffic, in its general effects, is '*intensely mischievous to every branch of trade.*'

COTTON GOODS AND THE OPIUM TRADE.

By REV. GOODEVE MABBS,

Organizing Secretary to the Society for the Suppression of the Opium Trade.

The population of China is alleged to be 400 millions, or one-third of the inhabitants of the globe. China ought, therefore, to afford one of the largest markets in the world for British exports. But instead of this, as a matter of fact, our China trade is relatively of infinitesimal proportions. The figures are as follows:—

    Exports to China, 1879   .   .   .   .   £8,268,413.
    Exports to China, 1880   .   .   .   .   9,482,822.

CHINESE MERCHANTS.

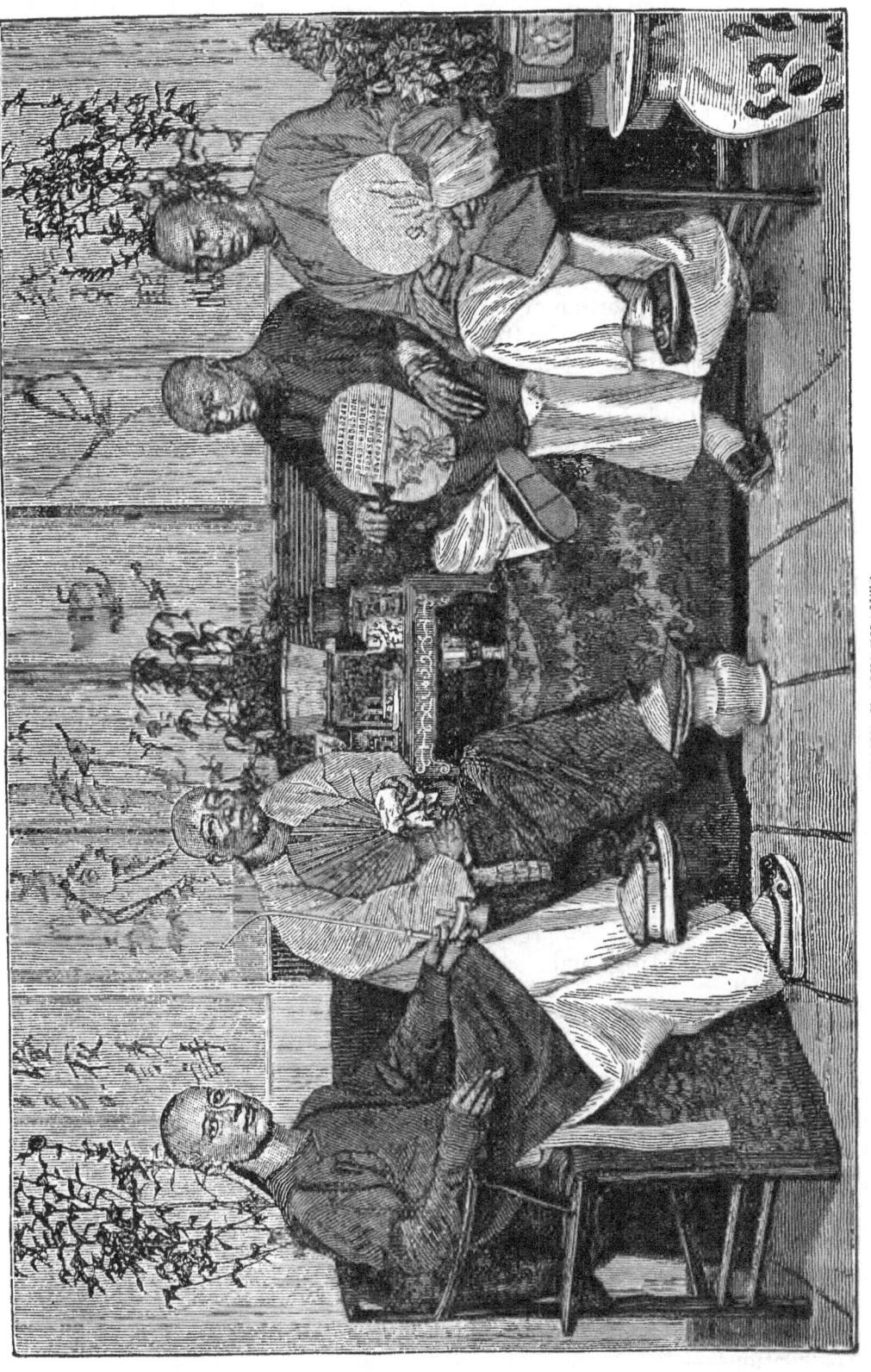

These show an increase for the year of nearly one million and a quarter compared with nine millions and three-quarters increase in India. But again, 1879 was not a prosperous year for trade with China as compared with several preceding years. From 1869 to 1872 the value of British exports to China (including in all cases Hong-Kong and Macao) ranged between nine millions and nearly ten millions sterling. In the first of those years it was £9,240,161. So that going back, as before, over a period of twelve years, we get an increase in 1880 of less than a quarter of a million sterling, being at the rate of less than three per cent. as compared with about seventy-three per cent. in India. Taking the population of China at 300 millions, instead of 400 millions, the exports in 1880 gave a proportion of slightly over 7d. per head. During the same year the Chinese at the treaty ports—that is, at the only channels of trade open to us—were paying to the opium merchants from £14,000,000 to £16,000,000 for opium.

If it be contended that the fact of India being governed by ourselves makes the comparison with China scarcely fair to the latter, let us take the case of the neighbouring country, Japan, from which opium is excluded by treaty, made shortly after that of Tientsin, by which we forced opium upon China. The population of Japan is stated to be about 36,000,000. The exports from Great Britain for 1879 and 1880 are as follows:—1879, £2,997,522; 1880, £3,813,397. This gives an increase of considerably over three-quarters of a million; but in 1869 these exports amounted to £1,595,868, so that during the last twelve years the increase has been nearly two millions and a quarter sterling, or at the rate of 150 per cent.

In order that it may be seen that India and Japan are not selected for comparison with China because they are exceptionally favourable for that purpose, I subjoin a table of eight of the countries with which our principal trade is carried on:—

	Imports from England. £	Value per Head. £ s. d.	Rate of Increase in 12 years.
Australia	18,748,000	6 11 6¼	30 p.c.
Cape of Good Hope and Natal	7,206,000	4 9 6	3.83 p.c.
West Indies	2,451,662	1 19 2½	16 p.c.[1]
British N. America	8,516,019	1 19 1½	41 p.c.
United States	37,954,192	0 14 7	41 p.c.
India	32,028,055	0 2 6	73 p.c.
Japan	3,813,397	0 2 1	150 p.c.
China, with Hong-Kong and Macao	8,842,509	0 0 7	3 p.c.[1]

It will thus be seen that China stands proportionally at the very bottom of the list.

The following table applies exclusively to the values of cotton goods exported from Great Britain, and the rate per head for the various populations:—

[1] Nearly.

	£	Per Head.
		s. d.
Australia	1,782,778	12 6
Cape of Good Hope and Natal.	609,486	7 7
West Indies	562,519	9 0
British North America	918,024	4 2½
United States	3,698,268	1 5
India	21,093,267	1 8
Japan	2,007,860	1 1¼
China, with Hong-Kong and Macao	6,178,344	0 4½

If commercial Manchester will address itself to finding a satisfactory solution to the question, Why is it that China, instead of being, as it ought to be, the largest and best market for British imports, is relatively one of the worst? it will find reason to welcome the movement for the suppression of the opium trade as an ally, instead of being jealous of it as at present. . . . Depend upon it, there is no greater barrier, both politically and economically, to the extension of British trade with China than our British Indian opium trade. The seven or eight millions of revenue which India obtains from the traffic really comes out of the till of the British manufacturer and from the resources of the British people. How long will Englishmen submit to this?—*Extract from letter to the Editor of the 'Manchester Guardian.'*

London Bankers on the Opium Trade.

In a Letter to the Chambers of Commerce.

We lay stress on this outstanding fact, that English industry is practically shut out from the market which of all others seems to offer the greatest possibilities of increase and expansion; and this not from any unwillingness on the part of the Government or people of China to receive our manufactures, but through the calamitous operation of a monopoly which exists for the sake of bringing in revenue to the Indian Exchequer. The purchasing power of China seems paralyzed by the opium trade, whilst the Indian budget rests upon a basis which must give way the moment China is strong enough to assert herself.

Mr. S. Manders

On Trade with China.

It was a legitimate expectation, cherished from the beginning of our intercourse with China, that an immense trade would ultimately spring up between that country on the one hand, and England and India on the other. But, after a hundred years of intercourse, what are the facts? In 1874, with twenty-one seaports open to us, in addition to the possession of Hong-Kong, England sent to China, with its 400 millions of inhabitants (nearly one-third of the human race), less than £8,000,000 worth of goods, out of a total export to all countries of £250,000,000, that is, less than fourpence per head per annum of its population; while the Australian Colonies, with only four millions of people, took £14,000,000 worth of our goods, or just £3, 10s. per head per annum.

Dr. Dudgeon

ON THE COMMERCIAL LOSS TO ENGLAND CAUSED BY THE OPIUM TRADE.

The commerce and manufactures of our country are seriously affected by the trade, so much so that, in one sense, we might say Great Britain pays over eight millions annually to India. We and the Chinese are the sufferers by the trade. . . . Were this traffic abolished, there is almost nothing in the way of progress in the opening up of the country and facilitating of trade that they are not, I believe, prepared to do.

THE OPIUM TRADE, AS NOW CARRIED ON, A NATIONAL SIN, WHICH MUST BRING RETRIBUTION.

Dr. Norman Macleod

ON THE PUNISHMENT OF NATIONAL SIN.

It is perhaps true that to connect the sufferings of individuals or of nations with their sins may be a very difficult task now-a-days, and one in which the vision of the wisest 'seer' may be perverted by the darkness of ignorance and the bias of his own prejudices or passion. It may also be alleged that, so far as we can discover, God now leaves men to the sole operation of His natural laws, to be punished by the consequences of disobedience to them. . . .

And what though God be ruling over us and revealing His will to us by general laws; what though we can no more discern the supernatural, if His government be supernatural, and not eminently mortal! Are we not taught by Scripture that God can in His own way and time, now as ever, and by fitting instrumentalities, visit the earth with judgments, and thereby carry out His holy purposes? Verily though 'the natural man' may see the natural only, yet the 'spiritual man' can see a living God also, if not in, yet from His working; a God who, in perfect harmony with all law, can, in the world of matter and of mind, touch far-off springs of power, by which forces may be either produced or held in check, so as to do His will. He surely can give to or withhold from man wisdom, skill, genius, power; and in many ways, which no human eye can foresee, may reward well-doing or punish wrong-doing. He can punish the wicked by even letting him 'eat of the fruit of his own ways, and be filled with his own devices.' And He can humble the pride of wealth, punish its selfish expenditure, and destroy the godless boasting of commercial prosperity, by the action of laws which can affect the treasures of gold and silver, through other treasuries known to Himself alone, such as 'the treasuries of the snow and of the hail, which He hath reserved to Himself against the day of trouble;' and by rain poured down or withheld from His secret laboratory, He can make the exchanges of the world to tremble or rejoice.—*From Sermon preached by Dr. Norman Macleod, published at the Queen's command, and also by her command dedicated to Her Majesty.*

Sir Arthur Cotton

ON RETRIBUTION FOR NATIONAL SIN.

When the American Government passed the fugitive slave law, and so sealed their own condemnation, Garfield said (how terribly true!) 'A covenant with death, and an agreement with hell, that will destroy the authors of it. The cry of the oppressed and down-trodden will appeal to the Almighty for retribution, like the blood of Abel. The lightning of divine wrath will shiver the old gnarled tree of slavery, leaving neither root nor branch.' And on the same subject of slavery, Lincoln said, 'What if every drop of blood drawn by the lash from the slave is paid for by blood drawn by the sword!' etc. These words also were exactly fulfilled. If we refuse to hear what God has thus declared in the civil war to all the world, what can we expect but that He will speak yet louder to us, upon whom as a nation He has heaped up such favours as no nation ever received?—*Letter to the Anti-Opium Society, by Sir Arthur Cotton.*

The late M‘Leod Wylie, Esq.,

ON NATIONAL SIN AND ITS PENALTY.

It must not be supposed that any Government can continue such a course as ours with impunity. 'God is not mocked.' In May 1839, our quarrel with China respecting the conduct of British subjects in reference to opium-smuggling was first brought to the test of arms, and troops and vessels were sent from India in the course of that year to aid Her Majesty's forces. In May 1840 commenced those risings against our power in Affghanistan which ended in the defeat and massacre of the entire British army, and a blow to our influence in India and Central Asia from which we have never recovered.

At the commencement of 1857, a quarrel, arising out of our protection of one of the smuggling-lorchas, was brought to the same test; we bombarded Canton, and the British nation, at a general election, enthusiastically ratified the policy of Government, and a large expedition, with an enormous amount of the munitions of war, was despatched 'to vindicate our honour.' Before that expedition could reach China, there burst forth in India a more terrible insurrection than has been known in modern history, and our formidable armament had to be diverted with all speed for the preservation of our Indian Empire. . . .

As the Spaniards and Portuguese carried to South America a corrupted Christianity, and in wickedness proved themselves worse than the heathen, so we in China are exhibiting, not love of our neighbour, but the most hateful selfishness, and are sowing the seeds of a blight and woe such as fell on the followers of the conquerors of Mexico and Peru. But if as a nation we will now redress this mighty wrong,—if we will now honestly set ourselves to the noble work of purging our national reputation from the stain of this disgrace,—if we will now at length discharge our solemn duty, and resolve, whatever may be the cost, that Britain shall no longer be guilty of hastening the temporal and eternal ruin of the millions of China, can it be doubted that God will bless us, and that we shall find, in giving up our five millions a year, that 'He is able to give us much more than this'? We may doubt how we can best accomplish our benevolent design, but our way will certainly be made plain, and the national recompense will be speedy and abundant.—*From Notes on the Opium Question by the late M'Leod Wylie, Esq., of Calcutta.*

CARDINAL MANNING

ON THE DANGER OF PERSISTING IN OUR OPIUM POLICY.

It seems to me manifest that if we deliberately, with our eyes open, persist in this course, we are preparing for ourselves a castigation which may come even from human hands. We despise the southern Chinese as an unwarlike people. What are the northern, and what are the western provinces of China? What are those armies that went forth the other day into the centre of Asia and met the Russian force? There is a power in China which one day may raise itself up, before which our great imperial army may find that it has a heavy task to do.

But more than this; there is a great empire that is hovering upon the frontiers of China, on the Amoor river, on the north and on the west, and on our north-west of India; and who knows that the scourge may not be there preparing for us if we alienate the Oriental races—if we make them distrust us—if we teach them to regard us as the destroyers of all that is dear to them—if they see that we are trading for money—that we are not controlled, I will not say by our Christianity, but by moral laws?

The member for South Durham the other day, instead of saying, 'Christian and international morality,' might have used the formula of our old jurists, 'The law of nature and of nations;' for it is a crime against the law of nations to poison a neighbouring people. If we go on so, the day may not be far distant when there will come the chastisement, and we shall deserve it.

The other day, a statesman worthy of the name—one of the leaders of our great political parties—in answer to some one who said, 'By what right do we hold India?' replied, 'By the divine right of good government.' That divine right of good government, as long as we persevere in justice, will avail. If we violate it, we tear up our imperial titles. Mighty as our will may be—and mighty indeed it is, for the British Empire is now in the zenith of its power—yet over the tumultuous waves of human wills there is one Sovereign Will that reigns. If we violate it, its judgment may come slowly, but its judgment will come surely at the last.—*Speech at the Mansion House Meeting on the Opium Question.*

PROTEST OF THE LATE R. MONTGOMERY MARTIN, ESQ.,

A Member of Her Majesty's Legislative Council at Hong-Kong.

In 1844, twenty opium-smoking shops were licensed in Hong-Kong in the name of Her Majesty the Queen of England. Mr. Montgomery Martin, who was at that time *Her Majesty's Treasurer for the Colonial, Consular, and Diplomatic Services in China, and a Member of Her Majesty's Legislative Council at Hong-Kong*, endeavoured in vain to prevent this being done, and put on record his protest, which was dated 'Council Room, Hong-Kong, November 26, 1844.'

In an official report to Her Majesty's Government, published two or three years later, Mr. Martin gave a singularly clear statement of the opium question in a chapter headed, 'Opium: Progress and Extent of Consumption; Individual and National Effects; Imperial Edicts; Denunciation by the Government; its Seizure and Destruction; State of the Traffic, and Unchristian Conduct of England.'

Mr. Martin closed his report with a very solemn and powerful appeal, from which the following is taken :—

OUR CAREER OF INIQUITY IN CHINA.

To dwell more on this distressing theme would be unnecessary; if the facts herein stated will not awaken the minds of those who *call themselves Christians in England*, neither would they hear 'although one rose from the dead.' It would be contrary to the admitted order of Divine Providence to suppose that such a career of iniquity as we have been pursuing in China, can bring with it any blessing. If there be a Supreme Being—the Creator of the universe and of man—*if He be a God of justice*, and have any regard for the creatures He has made, it is not possible to contend that He can view with indifference the commission of crimes, such as the previous pages incontestably establish.

AS A NATION SOWS, SO IT MUST REAP.

The grossest idolater admits and practically recognises the truth of this principle. Those who have the slightest belief in the Jewish and Christian Testaments, must, at least with their lips, acknowledge that the Creator and Preserver of mankind has, by example and precept, established most conclusively the retributive decree, that *as a nation sows so it must reap*. Can England reasonably expect peace and plenty at home when she is scattering poison and pestilence abroad? Can she, without hypocrisy, consecrate churches, and ordain ministers of a Christian faith, while her rulers and governors are licensing opium hells, and appointing supervisors to extract the largest amount of profit from the iniquity therein perpetrated?

UNPARALLELED WICKEDNESS.

Is Christianity a name, or is it a principle? What an abomination it must be in the sight of a great and good Deity to behold national prayers offered to Him to avert dispensation of calamity, while the very nation that is offering them is *daily inflicting destitution and death on more than three millions of our fellow-creatures!* Thus impiously seeking relief from its own suffering, while recklessly spreading sorrow, vice, and crime among myriads of mankind! The records of wickedness since the world was created, furnish no parallel to the wholesale murders which the British nation have been, and still are, hourly committing in China. Neither are they committing this awful destruction of human beings in ignorance. There never was a question on which our Parliament concurred more unanimously than on the iniquity of the opium trade; no senator ventured to say that that good man Lord Ashley has exaggerated in the slightest degree the magnitude of the evils which his lordship implored, with an eloquence heightened by piety, the Legislature to correct. On the contrary, the assembled representatives of the nation, men of all parties, ministers and ex-ministers, concurred with the noble lord in the enormity of the crime we were perpetrating, deplored its continued existence, and promised its correction.

PROGRESS IN EVIL-DOING.

What has been done since on the subject? Have we simply remained passive, and allowed the crimes and the murders caused by the opium trade to go on silently, unnoticed and unapproved by Her Majesty's Government? We cannot even allege the poor miserable plea of winking as a Government against a crime which it is pretended could not be checked. On the contrary, the representative of Queen Victoria has recently converted the small barren rock which we occupy on the coast of China into a vast 'opium-smoking shop;' he has made it the 'Gehenna of the waters,' where iniquities which it is pollution to name can not only be perpetrated with impunity, but are absolutely *licensed* in the name of our gracious sovereign, and protected by the titled representative of Her Majesty.

Better—far better—infinitely better—abjure the name of Christianity, call ourselves heathens, idolaters of the '*golden* calf,' worshippers of the 'evil one.'

Let us do this, and we have then a principle for our guide, the acquisition of money at any cost, at any sacrifice. Why, the 'slave trade' was merciful compared to the 'opium trade.' We did not destroy the bodies of the Africans, for it was our immediate interest to keep them alive; we did not *debase their natures, corrupt their minds,* nor *destroy their souls.* But the opium-seller slays the body after he has corrupted, degraded, and annihilated the moral being of unhappy sinners, while every hour is bringing new victims to a Moloch which knows no satiety, and where the English murderer and the Chinese suicide vie with each other in offerings at his shrine.

No blessing can be vouchsafed to England while this national crime is daily calling to Heaven for vengeance; none of the millions of mere nominal Christians who throng our churches one day in the week, can expect to prosper in their worldly callings, while they are silently abetting an awful crime, which no sophistry can palliate, no ingenuity refute.

We stand convicted before the nations of the world, as well as before an Omniscient Deity, from whom nothing can be hidden, as a Government and people actively and legally engaged in the perpetration of murder and desolation, on a scale of such magnitude as to defy calculation. Disguise it as we may, this is the naked truth,—this is the damning fact, which no water will obliterate.

We are all involved in the guilt, and participants, even by our silence, in a sin which, if not rooted out, must ere long bring on us that Divine vengeance, which, though slow, is sure, and never invoked in vain.

Finally, this report is dedicated (by gracious permission) to the Sovereign of the British nation, with an earnest prayer that the Almighty—by whose authority 'kings reign and princes decree justice'—may influence the councils of Her Majesty to do that which is right in the sight of Him who declareth that 'they who set their heart on their iniquity will have the reward of their doings.'—*From 'China: Political, Commercial, and Social;' in an official report to Her Majesty's Government.*

LIEUTENANT-GENERAL SIR ARTHUR COTTON, K.C.S.I.,

ON THE OPIUM QUESTION.

Sir Arthur Cotton's long connection with India gives weight to his opinion. For the information of any who may not be acquainted with his valuable services in India, we may quote the words of Sir Richard Temple, who says :—' Of the many benefactors of India in recent times, there are few who have done more material good than Sir Arthur Cotton during this generation,' and that ' his name will be handed down to the grateful remembrance of posterity ' (*India in* 1880, by Sir Richard Temple, Bart., late Governor of Bombay, Lieutenant-Governor of Bengal, and Finance Minister of India).

DORKING, *May* 6, 1882.

MY DEAR SIR,—I should be greatly obliged to you if you could allow me to add my own particular views on the opium question to your pamphlet on the subject.

In the course of my sixty years' connection with India, I have come to some conclusions, the result of actual experience, which bear in a particular manner upon the subject, and which certainly answer the main arguments of those who insist upon our continuing this trading upon the sins and miseries of the greatest nation in the world, in respect of population, on the ground of our needing the money.

But before touching upon these points, it is essential that I insist upon the great fundamental point, which is quite independent of all secondary considerations. My foundation is this, 'Be not deceived; God is not mocked; for whatsoever a man (or nation) soweth, that shall he also reap.' No power on earth can escape from this sentence. The harvest of money which we are at present reaping is not the harvest of this trade.

The burglar congratulates himself on the contents of the purse, which he looks upon as his harvest. But he learns what is really the harvest, when he finds himself commencing ten years' hard labour in gaol without remuneration, aggravated by an accusing conscience without one hope. The Americans thought their harvest was a few millions a year, extracted by the lash and secured by immeasurable crimes; but the real harvest was the loss of a thousand millions of money, and a million of their most valuable lives, and many millions of bereaved fathers, mothers, brothers, sisters, friends, and dependants of all kinds. This was their proper harvest. What they sowed they also reaped. Every drop of blood drawn by the lash was, as Lincoln said, paid for by a bucketful drawn by the sword.

We thus learn that there is a God in heaven, a God who is not mocked. We have already reaped in famines and mutiny, but assuredly all this is nothing to what is before us, if, in the face of God's dealings with America, and with ourselves, we persist in what is bringing utter destruction upon so many millions in China.

Our shutting our own eyes to the wrong we are doing won't the least defer this harvest. All the subtle arguings about our need of the money, the supply of opium by other countries, the half-heartedness of the Chinese authorities, etc., won't affect the results a hair's-breadth. The question is between us and God. 'Whatsoever a man soweth, that shall he also reap,' without the smallest diminution in consequence of what others may do, even the Chinese themselves.

But now with reference to the argument that we cannot do without this revenue from opium. My answer is, that it is utterly false. God has been pleased so to prosper our rule in India, that she is at this moment perfectly independent of this accursed money; and if we persist in the iniquity of obtaining revenue by forcing opium upon China, it must be in the face of the abundant prosperity which God has granted to India through our means. He is now acknowledging our, in the main, faithful, upright, laborious rule of India, by such a progress in material prosperity as never was seen in any country in the world, and I can see no cloud overhanging our rule there, except this astonishing national crime.

The budget just published shows a clear large surplus of *ordinary* revenue over *ordinary* expenditure, exclusive of opium, and of the net returns from public works. The accounts of public works show a surplus of one million above the interest of the capital invested. But this account includes the loss upon the Indus railways, which cost twenty millions, and which are strategic and do not belong to the category of ordinary investments; they belong to the class of wars, famines, etc., which are extraordinary expenditures, and should be a permanent charge upon the country, and not a charge upon the present generation. On these railways there is a net loss of about half a million a year, I calculate, leaving a clear surplus of one and a half million upon the proper ordinary public works investments.

This is an astonishing result, when we remember that not one of these works is yet fully developed. A large proportion of them have only lately been opened, and are not yielding a quarter of their ultimate returns, some not even a tenth part, and some are not yet opened. When all these are in extensive operation, it is certain that the returns will exceed the present amount by several millions. The two most costly works are at this moment returning ten per cent. net. But, again, these are only the direct returns in money. They do not include the indirect returns in the shape of ordinary taxes from the increased wealth of the people. Thus, while the Godavery irrigation returns £180,000 in water rates on an expenditure of £800,000, the increase of the whole revenue of the district is £400,000.

The recent budget does at last acknowledge the flourishing state of Indian finance, and it takes off three millions of taxes; and, by the way, this, to the honour of the present rule, entirely to the relief of the working-classes. But in spite of all the subtle arguments of great statesmen, honesty is the best policy. Most assuredly, the very first step to the thorough establishment of the finances on the soundest foundation, is the removal of this vile opium revenue. Happily nothing in the world is easier than to stop it. A field of poppies can't be concealed like a still, and the immediate and absolute prohibition of their cultivation can be carried out at once, though, of course, as in the case of slavery, many minor questions dependent upon it will have to be settled.

The points I insist upon are,—(1) the ordinary revenue is now in excess of the ordinary expenditure, independent of the opium revenue; (2) the extraordinary expenditure, that is, the cost of wars, famines, strategic works, etc., ought not to be laid upon the present generation, but be provided for by loans, *as they are in every other country;* (3) that we have now overwhelming proof, in the results of the present public works, that by the extension of such works we can abundantly provide for the interest, and even the gradual paying off of the principal, of any probable future extraordinary expenditure, provided only we don't provoke God to send us calamities beyond all calculation, and compel us, as He has done the United States, to lay on additional taxes, to the amount of fifty millions a year, to pay their slavery bill. How easily He can send a war or a mutiny, or at least a famine that will in a year sweep away all the millions we have made by this horrible trade !

It is quite certain that the present works will soon pay four or five millions a year above their interest, and that another hundred millions laid out in a similar manner would yield five millions a year more, above interest, in direct returns, besides the increase of ordinary taxes due to the increased income of the country from those works.

(4) The whole value of the opium crop per acre is 15 lbs. at $8\frac{1}{2}$ rupees (1200 rupees per chest of 140 lbs.), or 127 rupees; the sum stated by a local official in Behar to be the *net profit* to the ryot on an acre of sugar, making the value of the latter crop at least 200 rupees, *so that the loss to India by the growth of opium in place of sugar* is at least £7 per acre on 800,000 acres, or $5\frac{1}{2}$ millions *annually.* These are the essential points in the financial part of the question.

I *must* add, What conceivable right have we to force upon another country the principles upon which she shall conduct her internal affairs? Why don't we treat with China as we do with France or the United States, respecting our external trade with her, and leave her to order her internal trade as she chooses ? But now our threats are mere bluster. We are perfectly powerless in the matter; no Government of England would dare for a moment to hint at another opium war. China has nothing to do but to prohibit instantly the importation of opium, and we must accept her decision. She is most assuredly preparing to do this, and there is nothing whatever to prevent her doing it at this moment.

A gentleman of property lately said to me, 'Can you tell me anything about this opium question? It appears to me it must be terribly wrong to make money by forcing this evil upon another nation.' I am confident that this gentleman was only the representative of the great mass of the people of England, and that nothing is wanting but information to rouse the whole body of the nation, and to bring such a hurricane of public opinion upon the authorities as will sweep away every thought of attempting to continue this inconceivable national crime.

Who in England would not be horrified—even Sir G. Birdwood and Sir R. Alcock themselves—at the thought of making money by introducing opium into the families of their friends and neighbours, or fellow-workmen, with the certainty of bringing upon them incalculable misery? How much more to force it by tons upon a nation of four hundred millions, where already millions of families have been desolated beyond recovery!—Believe me, ever yours,

ARTHUR COTTON.

B. Broomhall, Esq.

IMPORTANT TESTIMONIES.

ARCHBISHOP OF CANTERBURY.

I have, after very serious consideration, come to the conclusion that the time has arrived when we ought most distinctly to state our opinion, that the course at present pursued by the Government in relation to this matter is one which ought to be abandoned at all costs.—*Speech at the Mansion House.*

THE ARCHBISHOP OF YORK

ON THE OPIUM TRADE.

We say that it is a wrong thing from first to last. We say that it is a disgrace and a shame to this country that a heathen people should have had to ask us to hold our hands and not to force the opium upon them, and that we, as a Christian people, should refuse to hold our hand, and with fire and sword make them take this deadly drug, which they were willing to abandon. I don't excuse myself for not having attended to this subject before. . . . We have now got firm hold of this subject, and I should think ill of the human mind if we let it go before we had mastered it, and dealt it such a blow that it shall never recover. . . .

This is a question affecting the whole of the human race for whom Christ died. It affects this great country in its honour and its consistency; it affects the population of China more vitally still. It affects all manufactures, because I am told that it is an established fact that the exports of every class are hindered by this difficulty about the opium question. There is hardly a class in this country, or remotely connected with this country, which is not affected by this question, and we, as ministers of religion, dear friends, are especially bound to it. We are bound by the example of One who went about the world doing good, and if we go about the world doing evil we are not only not with Him, but we are against Him, and He will, according to His law, cast us out. He loves all the people of the world alike, and we can't sit down, as some statesmen have done, by saying, 'Oh, we would abolish this trade if we could, but then consider the revenue.' Words like those have occurred in speeches, and even in public documents put forth in this country. We, as Christian ministers, have nothing to do with that; *though the whole of the revenue of India, from end to end, depended entirely on the opium traffic, if it is a sinful and wrong traffic, we are bound to protest against it,* and to seek other ways in which revenue of some sort can be supplied.

It is not a matter which we can afford any longer to treat with indifference; we will approach the Crown in every way that lies in our power, and we will express our opinion that the time has come to make the necessary arrangements for the suppression of this iniquitous traffic.

THE BISHOP OF MADRAS

ON ENGLAND WAKING UP TO THE SHAMEFUL WRONG OF FORCING OPIUM UPON CHINA.

The mind of England has at last awoke up to the shameful wrong which our Christian nation has for forty years past been inflicting upon China. Protectors of opium-smugglers, we forced the rulers of China, against their earnest protests, and with the powerful argument of our cannon, to open the ports for the admission of the drug, which was to besot and ruin the inhabitants of that vast empire by thousands, but would enrich the Indian exchequer. Missionaries and plenipotentiary have hitherto expostulated against the iniquity in vain.

The contribution from opium traffic of about eight millions of pounds every year to the Indian revenue, acting like a bribe, has promoted the avoidance of the question as to the righteousness or unrighteousness of England's conduct towards China. But now the public conscience is awake, and we may reasonably expect that China's wrongs at our hands will undergo full investigation; and that, if it should be found needful for righteousness' sake to sacrifice even the whole (which will, however, probably not be the case) of the opium revenue, our rulers will not hesitate to follow the dictates of justice and humanity, and suffer some inconvenience as retribution for the past injustice. And yet I am sure of this, that every sacrifice made in the name of God, either by an individual or by a nation, shall receive a full reward. We should never forget that reply of the prophet to Amaziah, the king of Judah, who had 'hired of the king of Israel a hundred thousand men for a hundred talents of silver; and there came a man of God to him, saying, O King, let not the army of Israel go with thee: for the Lord God is not with Israel. And Amaziah said to the man of God, But what shall we do for the hundred talents which I have given to the army of Israel? And the man of God answered, The Lord is able to give thee much more than this' (2 Chron. xxv. 7–9). By plenteous harvests, by increased and successful commerce, by averting wars, by a more widely extended spirit of honesty and industry, and in a thousand ways, great and small, God is able, if He will, so to add to the material prosperity of this empire, that whatever is required for its government shall be raised without extraordinary measures, without any murmuring of the people.—*Extract from Charge.*

THE EARL OF SHAFTESBURY

ON THE OPIUM TRAFFIC.

Speaking at a meeting of the China Inland Mission, his lordship said:—

Let every missionary, and every lay agent, and every woman, and every child refrain from being silent upon that question [the opium question]. The opium traffic is the greatest of modern abominations, and I believe that, unless it is corrected, it will bring upon this country of England one of the fiercest judgments that we have ever known.

THE LATE REV. DR. MORLEY PUNSHON,

In the report prepared and read by him at the meeting of the Wesleyan Missionary Society in Exeter Hall, said:—

All through China the brethren still deplore the blight of the opium traffic, *a greater national calamity than famine*, a calamity which enlightened heathen are urging a Christian nation, which first imposed it on them, to remove.

HENRY RICHARD, ESQ., M.P.,

ON THE OPIUM TRADE.

He had a firm conviction that no nation had ever been engaged in any business so absolutely indefensible on all moral and religious grounds as the traffic in opium. Even for the accursed slave trade something more plausible might be said than for the traffic in opium. It was said that by the slave trade good service was rendered to the African when he was carried away from the midst of pauperism and idolatry, and planted in the midst of a Christian community. But one thing only could be said for the traffic in opium, and that was that the Government wanted the revenue. It might be true that the opium which England was forcing upon the Chinese was spreading debauchery, demoralization, disease, and death among the Chinese—but there was the Indian revenue. It might be true that that traffic created an enormous amount of ill-will and heart-burning towards England on the part of the Chinese Government and the Chinese people, which had led at least to one war and might lead to another—but there was the Indian revenue. It might be true that that traffic constituted the most formidable of all obstacles against the effort to spread Christianity amongst the Chinese, as the missionaries testified—but then there was the Indian revenue. It might be true that it interfered with the development of other and more legitimate commerce—but there was the Indian revenue. It might be true that it dishonoured the character of England in the eyes of other nations, and prevented England protesting against the iniquitous practices of other nations—but there was the Indian revenue. But the question he wished to ask was, 'Are financial considerations for ever to overrule those of justice, morality, and religion?'

Mr. Bourke

Said in the House of Commons:—

The opium question had often been debated in the House, and he had never heard any one say aught in favour of the opium traffic from a moral point of view.

Resolutions passed at the Mansion House Meeting,

Held by invitation of the Right Hon. the Lord Mayor, on Friday, October 21st, 1881.

1. That in the opinion of this meeting the opium trade, as now carried on between India and China, is opposed alike to Christian and international morality and to the commercial interests of this country.
2. That in the opinion of this meeting it is the duty of this country, not only to put an end to the opium trade as now conducted, but to withdraw all encouragement from the growth of the poppy in India, except for strictly medicinal purposes, and to support the Chinese Government in its efforts to suppress the traffic.
3. That in the opinion of this meeting it will be the duty of this country to give such aid to the Government of India as may be found reasonable, in order to lessen the inconvenience resulting to its finances from the adoption of the policy advocated in the previous resolutions.
4. That in the opinion of this meeting the results of the sale of opium in British Burmah are a disgrace to our Government of India, and demand the most thorough and immediate remedy.
5. That a deputation from this meeting be appointed to lay before the Prime Minister the foregoing resolutions, and to press upon him the duty of adopting the policy therein approved; and that the Right Hon. the Lord Mayor, chairman of the meeting, and the Right Hon. the Earl of Shaftesbury, President of the Society, be requested to take the necessary steps to give effect to this resolution.

PARLIAMENTARY ACTION.

Notice of Motion by Sir J. W. Pease, M.P.,

In the Order Book of the House of Commons.

Mr. Joseph Pease,—Opium,—That an humble Address be presented to Her Majesty, praying that in the event of negotiations taking place between the Governments of Her Majesty and China, having reference to the duties levied on opium under the Treaty of Tien-tsin, the Government of Her Majesty will be pleased to intimate to the Government of China that in any such revision of that treaty the Government of China will be met as that of an independent State, having the full right to arrange its own import duties as may be deemed expedient.

The following letters in reference to petitions to Parliament in support of the above motion have been published :—

From His Grace the Archbishop of York.

BISHOPTHORPE, YORK, *March* 20, 1882.

MY DEAR SIR,—I sincerely hope that the clergy of the northern province, and especially those of my own diocese, may be induced to petition Parliament on the subject of the opium trade. The question is, whether a nation, convinced that the traffic in opium is injurious to the people, is to be free to make its own regulations as to the importation of the drug, or is to be coerced by a stronger nation, that has a good deal of opium to sell. China only asks for that power of self-government, in the matter of the opium traffic, which we exercise for ourselves in all matters. It is difficult to see any grounds for refusing such a right. That a Christian nation should be forcing the sale of a noxious drug upon a heathen nation that complains of and would reject it, is a sorry spectacle.—I am, yours very truly,

REV. STORRS TURNER. W. EBOR.

From the Right Rev. the Lord Bishop of Durham.

AUCKLAND CASTLE, BISHOP AUCKLAND,
March 23, 1882.

DEAR SIR,—The petitions in favour of Mr. Pease's motion have my cordial sympathy. It seems altogether unreasonable and unworthy of a Christian nation, that we should attempt to coerce China in the matter of the opium trade.

You are at liberty to make what use of this letter you please.

Yours faithfully,

REV. STORRS TURNER. J. B. DUNELM.

From the Right Rev. the Lord Bishop of Liverpool.

THE PALACE, LIVERPOOL, *March* 23, 1882.

SIR,—I shall be very glad if the clergy of the diocese of Liverpool are disposed to assist you in procuring petitions to the House of Commons against the opium traffic with China. I am convinced that such traffic is indefensible on moral grounds, and I think it ought to be stopped, like the slave trade in the West Indies, whatever the present sacrifice may be. 'The blessing of the Lord alone maketh rich, and He addeth no sorrow therewith.'—Yours faithfully,

To the SECRETARY. J. C. LIVERPOOL.

From the Right Rev. the Lord Bishop of Exeter.

The Palace, Exeter, *March* 25, 1882.

Sir,—I do not think it possible to defend our treatment of China. No nation has a right to compel another to take its goods by force of arms, still less to take what certainly may do much moral mischief, and what the weaker nation professes itself unwilling to receive on that very ground. We have no right whatever to force the Chinese to buy our opium. And the wrong is aggravated by the fact that we are Christians, and therefore doubly bound to act on high principles. Our conduct cannot but lower the Christian name in the eyes of all the heathen.

I sincerely hope that many of the clergy of this diocese will join in petitioning Parliament to put a stop to this scandalous injustice, and will induce others to join also. And you are quite at liberty to make use of this letter in any application you make to them.—Yours faithfully,

Rev. Storrs Turner. F. EXON.

HOW WE TEMPT THE CHINESE.

MAKING IT AS ATTRACTIVE AS POSSIBLE.

My own acquaintance with the subject dates from the year 1831, when in passing, by water, the chief opium magazine of the East India Company at Patna, I paid a visit to a friend who had charge of the scientific department of it. After he had led me through storey after storey, and gallery after gallery of the factory, with opium balls right and left, in tiers of shelves to the ceiling; upon my expressing amazement at an exhibition of opium, enough to supply the medical wants of the world for years, he replied nearly in these words: 'I see you are very innocent; these stores of opium have no such beneficent destination. It is all going to debauch the Chinese, and my duty is to maintain its smack as attractive to them as possible. Come to my laboratory.' There I saw broken balls of opium, procured, I understood, from China, by the Bengal government, as approved musters [samples] for imitation by the cultivators.—*From* 'The Traffic in Opium in the East' (p. 10), *by Julius Jeffrey, F.R.S. Extracted from the Appendix to his larger work,* 'The British Army in India.'

OPIUM IN EXCHANGE FOR TEA.

A THOUGHT FOR THE TEA-TABLE.

Let us look our position fairly in the face. China sends this country vast supplies of tea and of silk. If we trace *these* to their ultimate distribution, we shall find them bringing increased comfort and happiness to nearly every family in the United Kingdom. Our return for these valuable commodities is made chiefly in opium; and if we follow *that* article to the homes of its millions of consumers, we find that its mission is to debase and ruin, to lure its victims to a premature and utterly wretched end, and to plunge their families into destitution and misery.—*Rev. James Johnston.*

SIGNS OF PROGRESS.

On every hand there are indications of the awaking of the public mind to the importance of the opium question. The progress of public opinion on the subject is very remarkable, and should encourage to more vigorous effort all who are working for the suppression of our opium trade with China.

Of the many signs of progress the three following may be noted :—

I. THE ACTION OF THE GREAT RELIGIOUS BODIES OF ENGLAND.

Resolutions in condemnation of the opium trade have been passed in the most important representative meetings of the leading sections of the Christian Church, and petitions to Parliament have also been presented. Sir Edward Fry, in referring to this, says :—

'One petition was signed by Cardinal Manning and nearly all the Roman Catholic Bishops of England and Wales. The Convocation of the Province of York, after discussion, passed a strong resolution in condemnation of the trade. The Conference of the Wesleyans, the Synod of the Presbyterian Church of England, the General Assembly of the Free Church of Scotland, the Baptist Union, the Primitive Methodists, the Congregational Union, the Unitarians, and the Positivists, have all, like the Society of Friends, joined in petitions or resolutions to the like effect. If only these bodies should eagerly and zealously insist on effect being given to their resolutions, a great step will have been gained towards the ultimate solution of the question. This expression of opinion on the part of the religious bodies of England, new, I believe, as regards its generality, is a fact which may well encourage the efforts of all interested in the question.'

II. THE RESPONSE TO THE PROPOSAL TO RAISE A GUARANTEE FUND OF £25,000.

The support given to the proposal to raise a large fund for the purpose of carrying on with greater vigour the work of the Society for the Suppression of the Opium Trade, is an unmistakeable sign of progress. Some who are in earnest in the matter, and who feel that it is only needful for the public mind to be fully informed upon the question, to ensure that China shall no longer be compelled to admit our opium, have promised to the guarantee fund sums as under :

J. E. Wilson, Esq., J.P., £1000.
Sir J. W. Pease, Bart., M.P., £1000.
Arthur Albright, Esq., £500.
Arthur Pease, Esq., M.P., £500.
Samuel Smith, Esq., £500.
J. G. Barclay, £250.
J. C. Clayton, £250.

W. Fowler, Esq., M.P., £250.
Hugh Mason, Esq., M.P., £250.
Three Friends, £250.
Thomas Harvey, Esq., £100.
Peter Spence, Esq., £100.
Miss Fife, £100.
And many others from £1 to £50.

III. THE SIGNATURES TO THE MEMORIAL TO MR. GLADSTONE.

The memorial to Mr. Gladstone, imploring his 'powerful aid in setting right the relations between England and China as regards the opium trade, and so in removing a foul blot from our character as a civilised and Christian nation,' was signed by—

The Archbishops of Canterbury, York, and Dublin.

The Bishops of Durham, Carlisle, Exeter, Gloucester and Bristol, Hereford, Liverpool, Manchester, Norwich, Ripon, Salisbury, St. Albans, Winchester, Edinburgh, and Victoria.

Deans of St. Paul's and Canterbury.
Canons Gregory, Hoare, Stowell.

The President of the Wesleyan Conference (Rev. G. Osborn, D.D.).
The Chairman of the Congregational Union (Rev. Henry Allon, D.D.).
The President of the Baptist Union (Rev. Henry Dowson).
The Moderator of the Presbyterian Church in Ireland (Rev. W. Fleming Stevenson, D.D.).

Rev. Principal Brown, D.D. (Aberdeen); Rev. Principal Cairns, D.D. (Edinburgh); Rev. Principal Douglas, D.D. (Glasgow); Rev. Principal Newth, D.D. (London); Rev. Wm. Arthur, M.A.; Rev. T. Aveling, D.D.; Rev. Horatius Bonar, D.D.; Rev. Dawson Burns, M.A.; Rev. Thain Davidson, D.D.; Rev. J. Oswald Dykes, D.D.; Rev. Newman Hall, LL.B.; Rev. James Legge, D.D., Professor of Chinese, Oxford University; Rev. J. Kennedy, D.D.; Rev. Alex. Maclaren, D.D.; Rev. J. A. Macfadyen, M.A.; Rev. W. B. Pope, D.D.; Rev. John Stoughton, D.D.

Cardinal Manning. Duke of Westminster.
Earls of Shaftesbury and Cavan.
Lords—Ebury, Polwarth, Radstock.
Judges— Sir Ed. Fry; the late Sir R. Lush.

Members of Parliament—Wm. M'Arthur; J. W. Pease; Samuel Morley; W. S. Allen; John Barran; Hugh Birley; H. Broadhurst; W. S. Caine; C. Cameron; J. Cropper; J. Passmore Edwards; R. N. Fowler; W. Fowler; Theodore Fry; J. H. Kennaway; Hugh Mason; Arthur Pease; Henry Richard; W. Archdale; B. Armitage; W. C. Borlase; T. Burt; T. Chambers; J. C. Clark; J. J. Colman; Jesse Collings; J. Corbett; D. Davies; R. Davies; J. F. B. Firth; Lewis Fry; T. Green; J. Rowley Hill; W. Holmes; C. H. Hopwood; A. Illingworth; W. H. James; D. J. Jenkins; T. Lea; J. J. Leeman; A. M'Arthur; P. M'Lagan; C. M'Laren; C. H. Meldon; Arnold Morley; G. Palmer; W. S. Palmer; J. N. Richardson; P. Rylands; J. Simon; J. C. Stevenson; J. Stewart; A. M. Sullivan; T. H. Tillett; B. Whitworth; S. Williamson; J. Wilson; C. H. Wilson.
Lieutenant-General Sir Arthur Cotton, K.C.S.I.
Lieutenant-General Tremenheere, C.B.
Rev. Dr. Abbott, Head Master, City of London School.

Rev. Dr. Jex Blake, Head Master, Rugby School.
Rev. Dr. Butler, Head Master, Harrow School.
J. Agar, Esq., Lord Mayor of York.

Sir Edward Baines; Sir Thomas Charley, Q.C.; Sir Wm. Collins; Samuel Budgett, Esq., Bristol; John Cory, Esq., Cardiff; Professor Beesley, University College, London; Professor Leoni Levi, King's College, London; Professor Cowell, Cambridge; Professor Calderwood, Edinburgh; Professor Green, Oxford; Professor Geddes, Aberdeen; Professor King, Oxford; Rev. J. Percival, M.A., President of Trinity College, Oxford; Thomas Hughes, Esq., Q.C.; David M'Laren, Esq., J.P., D.L., Edinburgh; Donald Matheson, Esq.; James E. Mathieson, Esq.; J. C. Parry, Esq.; Joseph Sturge, Esq., Birmingham; Samuel Smith, Esq., Liverpool; S. D. Waddy, Esq., Q.C.; and many other persons of influence, including Presidents of Chambers of Commerce, Chairmen of School Boards, and thirty Mayors of Provincial towns.

CHINESE ILLUSTRATIONS OF THE OPIUM-SMOKER.

THE following illustrations by a Chinese artist are intended to represent different stages in the progress of the opium-smoker. The entire series, consisting of twelve sketches, have been beautifully coloured, and published with descriptive letterpress, by S. W. PARTRIDGE, 9 Paternoster Row, London, and may be had through any bookseller. Price 6d.

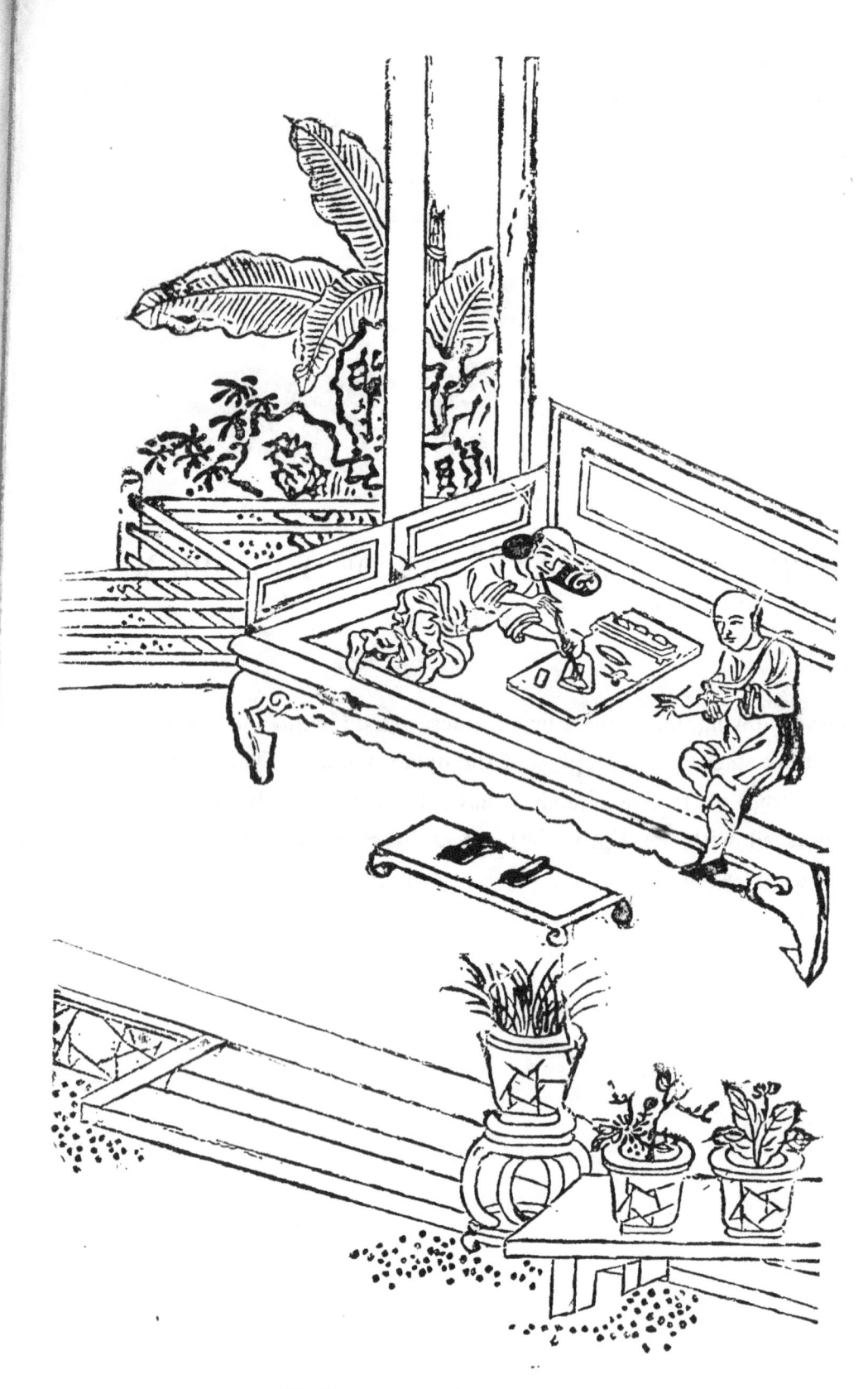

THE OPIUM-SMOKER'S FIRST PIPE.

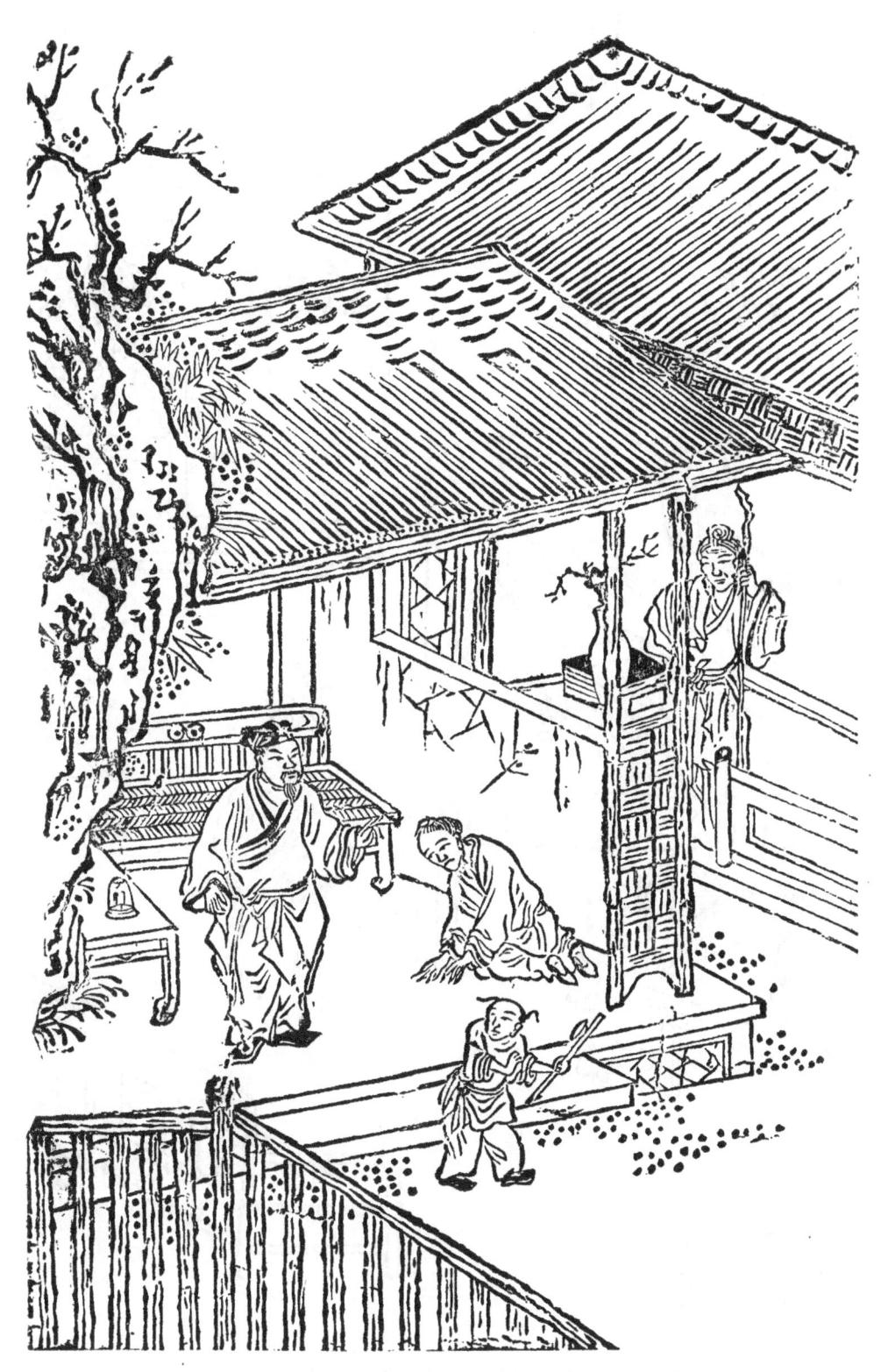

ENTREATED BY HIS FAMILY TO GIVE UP THE PIPE.

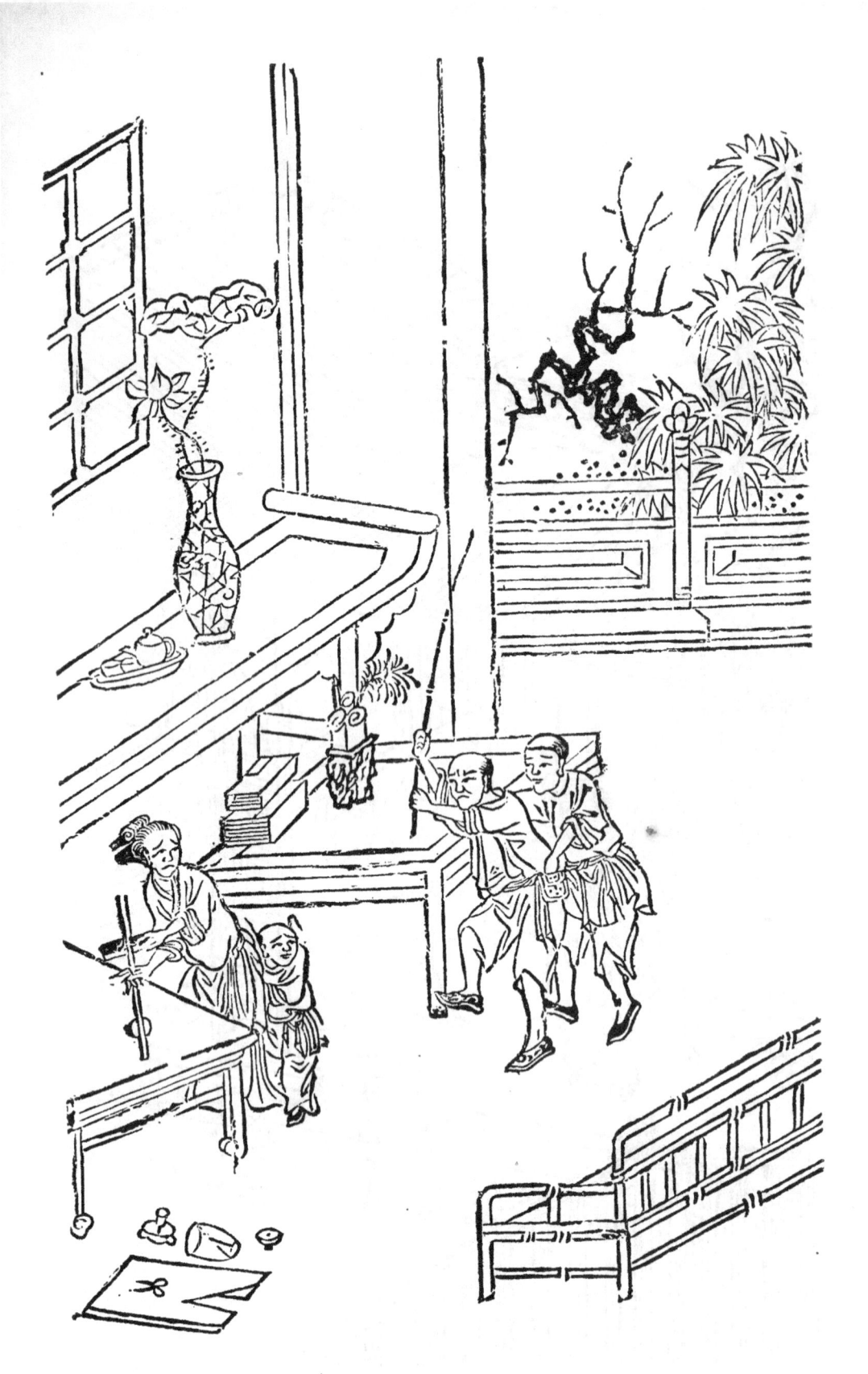

WIFE ATTEMPTS TO DESTROY HIS PIPE, ETC.

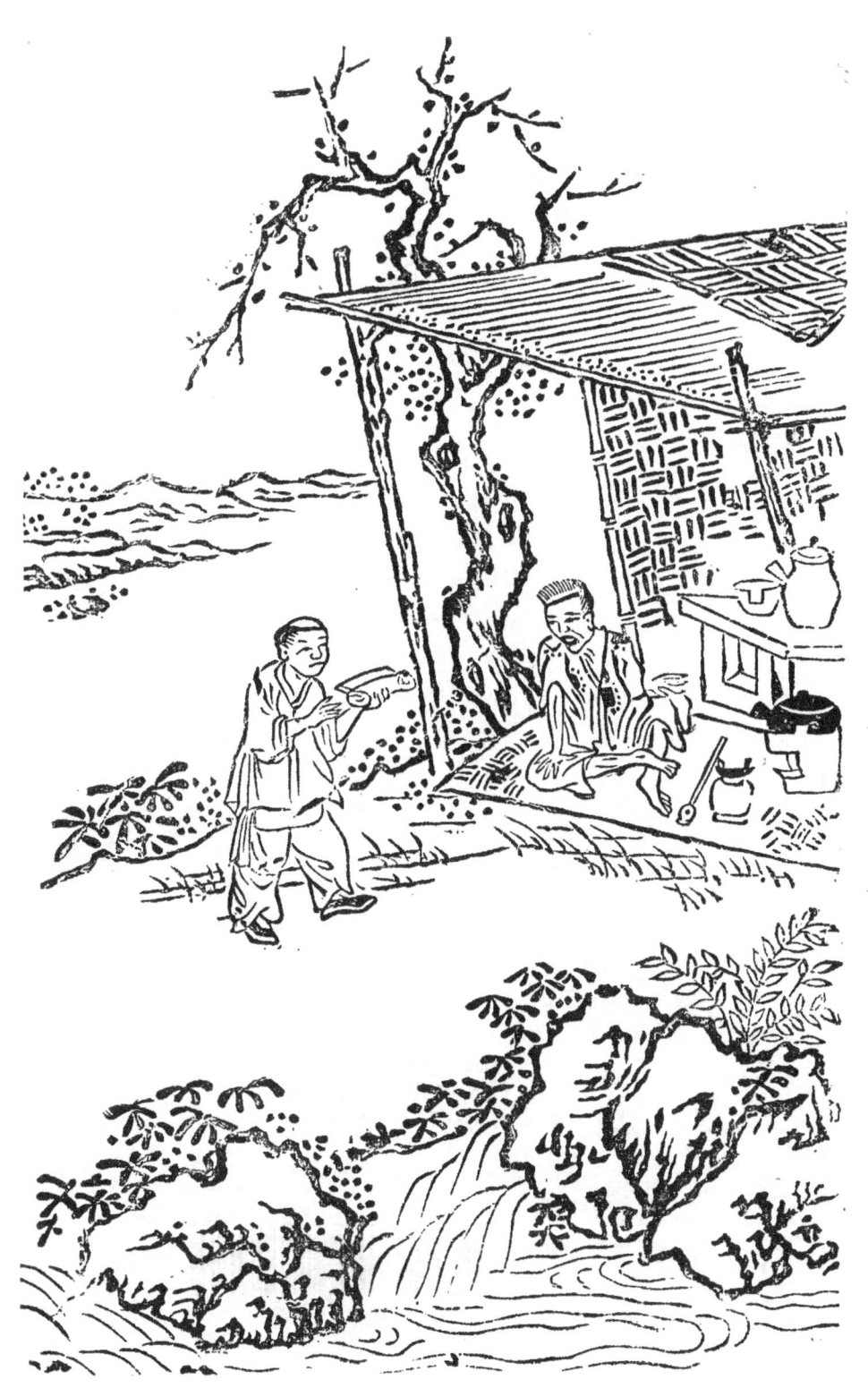

A HOUSELESS WANDERER.

Made in United States
North Haven, CT
30 December 2024